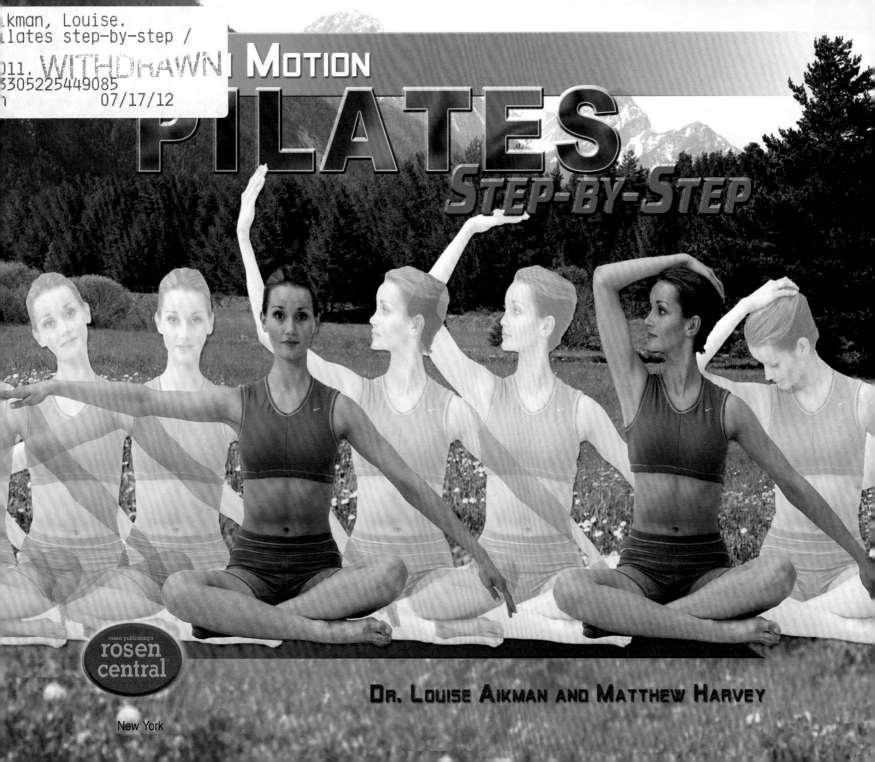

IN MOTION

PILATES
STEP-BY-STEP

rosen publishing's
rosen
central

DR. LOUISE AIKMAN AND MATTHEW HARVEY

New York

This edition published in 2011 by:

The Rosen Publishing Group, Inc.
29 East 21st Street
New York, NY 10010

Library of Congress Cataloging-in-Publication Data

Aikman, Louise.
Pilates step-by-step / Louise Aikman and Matthew Harvey.
    p. cm.—(Skills in motion)
Includes bibliographical references and index.
ISBN 978-1-4488-1549-4 (library binding)
1. Pilates method. I. Harvey, Matthew. II. Title.
RA781.4.A38 2011
613.7'192—dc22

                                                    2010007510

Manufactured in the United States of America

CPSIA Compliance Information: Batch #S10YA: For further information, contact Rosen Publishing, New York, New York, at 1-800-237-9932.

contents

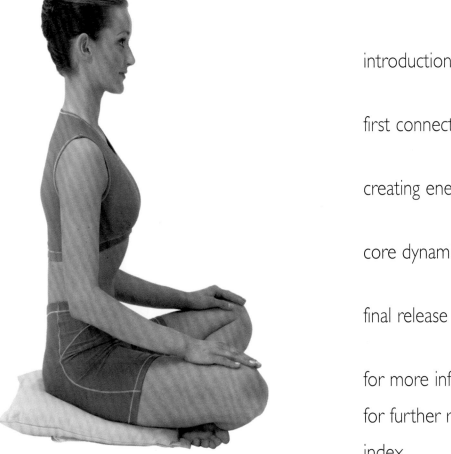

introduction

Although you may only recently have heard or read about Pilates, it has been in existence for about eighty years. Once dubbed "the fitness world's best kept secret," it remained relatively unknown because there were few instructors trained to teach it and even fewer studios with the equipment used for some of the exercises.

Over the last several years, the popularity of Pilates has grown beyond recognition, leading one writer to label it "the fastest growing global fitness trend."

You can now find Pilates matwork classes in most health clubs and public leisure centers, and specialized studios are opening up independently in clubs and spas. You may be offered Pilates-style exercises by your health care practitioner if you have a back problem, or you may be doing some Pilates already in the "core stability" part of your usual fitness class at the gym.

So what is it?

To get the most out of your Pilates class, or if you are using this book and practicing at home, you need to understand a little about the background of the Pilates system and the principles behind it. Developed by Joseph Pilates (1880–1967), the Pilates method is an interrelated system of exercises designed to challenge your strength, flexibility, and coordination. Joseph Pilates firmly believed that fitness was not just about developing and maintaining perfect, muscular bodies and gaining fitness and competitive performance, but a "unity of mind, body, and spirit."

Perhaps it is this philosophy as well as the benefits of the exercises themselves that account for people converting to his system in such numbers.

When you perform a Pilates exercise you are never just tightening one area of the body, stretching another, or mindlessly powering your way through a series of reps.

Each movement requires your full concentration as you train yourself to control your alignment and target your body's deeper muscles. As part of the process, you also have to learn to let go of the muscle tension that distorts your posture and your ability to perform the exercises correctly. To help achieve this, a flowing breathing pattern has to be mastered for each exercise.

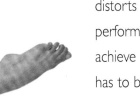

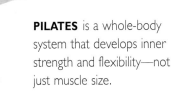

PILATES is a whole-body system that develops inner strength and flexibility—not just muscle size.

PRINCIPLES ARE PRINCIPLES...

In the years since his death, Joseph Pilates' original exercises have been developed by many teachers around the world, often making use of new knowledge that we have about how the body works and how to exercise effectively.

The following key principles still hold true, although each Pilates teacher has his or her own approach and may emphasize things a little differently depending on his or her experience and focus.

- **concentration**
- **control**
- **center**
- **alignment**
- **breathing**
- **flowing movement**

Understanding what each principle means will help you to get the most out of this book and your Pilates practice.

concentration and control

A famous quotation of Joseph Pilates reads "it is the mind that builds the body." Recent research seems to back this up. Using computer imaging, it is now possible to show that just thinking about moving a muscle sends a shower of impulses through the nervous system.

Pilates uses this "imaging" to get the most out of each movement. You have to be mindful, not mindless, when you do Pilates so, to help you, consider the following points before you begin:

- choose a time of day when you are least distracted or likely to be interrupted
- make sure the room is warm and that you have a comfortable mat to work on
- do not exercise if you have just eaten or are hungry— your concentration will be impaired
- if you choose to play music, pick something that will stay in the background without a strong beat
- whatever is bothering you—leave it behind. You will need all your attention for the exercises

Many Eastern systems believe this "one pointedness" is the key to self-development. Joseph Pilates was aware of this, but in building his own system, he focused on developing mental control by linking mind and body in a practical way, using breathing and visualization with each exercise. In a Pilates studio or class, the teacher will help you do this by using key words or images to give you the "visual flavor" or feel of the moves.

To help you do this at home, study the photographs and the text fo each exercise and try to picture each movement in your mind's eye before you begin. Visualize yourself performing the moves in the pictures and imagine the feeling of the muscles you will be using as indicated in the text

This "mental rehearsal" is important; it will help to get the correc muscles working (something a teacher would normally check for you by looking or feeling for muscle activity) and put a stop to other overworking. Bad posture and habits often cause muscles to work when they don't need to. Pilates encourages us to let go of old patterns so tha new and better ones can take their place.

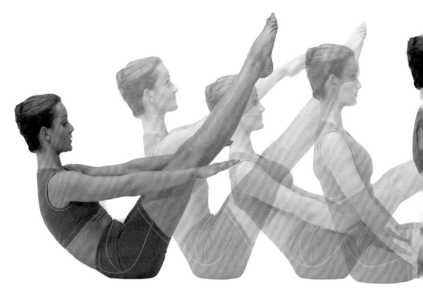

Joseph Pilates believed that movement should be controlled and subject to our will rather than our whim (or somebody else's). In typical fitness training, the "getting into" a move is often targeted more than the getting out. We pay attention as we load our muscles, but forget that how we unload them is just as important.

Pilates requires you to be aware of your body—how you are holding it, which muscles are about to be relaxed, and which are about to be activated—throughout each exercise.

Pilates stresses that the "eccentric" part of movement (returning to rest) is as important, perhaps even more important than the active, "concentric" part. When it comes to exercise, both need to be addressed.

This is why Pilates is often used as a key element in advanced fitness training or in rehabilitation programs after injury. Joseph Pilates seems to have predicted this, and you can benefit from his discoveries by paying attention to the following "technique" points:

● Practice how you get into and out of an exercise. For example, in a spine curl, how you curl out of the move is as crucial as how you curl up into it. Train your body not to slump or collapse out of an exercise, but return your spine to the mat or limbs back to the start position carefully.

● Practice an "arc of control"—give equal weight and attention to all parts of the exercise so you don't speed through the tougher parts. Your limbs are your levers, and you need to control their weight and direction of movement to gain the maximum benefit from the exercises.

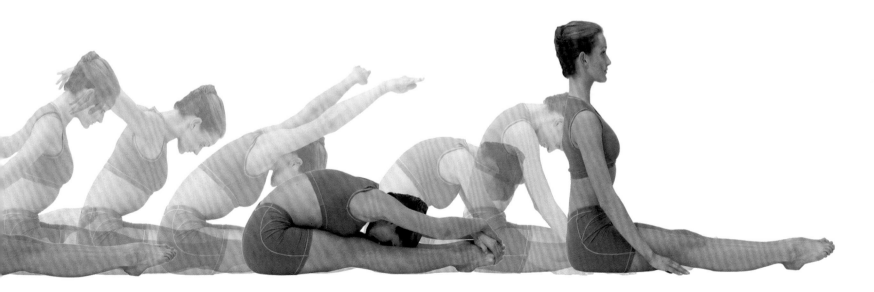

center and alignment

This is perhaps the most important Pilates principle, and the one responsible for many of the benefits claimed for the method. For Joseph Pilates the center (or "powerhouse," as he called it) was to be activated throughout each exercise. Pilates teachers often talk about creating a strong center from which movement can flow. What they mean by this is focusing on core muscles around the spine, the lower abdominals, and the pelvic floor to create a stable base for all movement.

Pilates himself advocated a bracing or pulling in of the abdominals. Most teachers now suggest a more gentle hollowing designed to target the deeper abdominals rather than the "six pack." The following exercise will help you achieve this. Try to practice it several times a day, first lying down and then sitting and standing.

Lying in relaxation position, place your hands on your lower abdomen. Breathe in gently, and as you breathe out, draw the lower part of your abdomen in toward your spine ("hollowing"). If your abdomen "kicks up" under your hands or bulges, you are working too hard—aim for a gentle tension like a drum skin being gradually tightened.

Use the breathing to help you (breathing out makes the hollowing or tightening easier to feel), and then practice holding the gentle contraction while you breathe quietly in and out. Now try this exercise standing and sitting. Once you master the basic abdominal contraction, you can put into your Pilates exercising—ideally this "pre-activation" should happen at the start of each exercise and run on quietly in the background while your other muscles coordinate the movements.

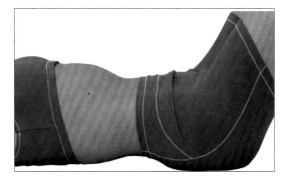

NEUTRAL The abdominals have been hollowed. Engaging the muscles around the spine, the lower abs and pelvic floor helps control the back's position.

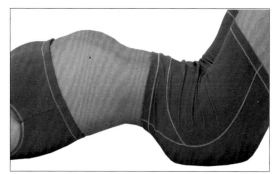

OVERARCHING Here, the shape and position of the back needs more abdominal work to bring it closer to "neutral." This position is not in neutral.

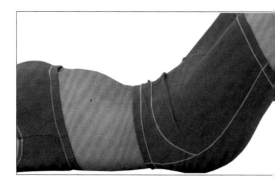

TUCKING UNDER Here, the neutral curve has been lost and the lower spine flattened into the mat. The spine is not in its neutral position.

Pilates requires you to multi-task. As you work through an exercise, you have to think not only about the muscles you are working (and not working), but also your overall body position.

Your alignment refers not only to the placement of your spine and limbs in a given exercise, but also your posture in daily life. Good posture relies on a series of gentle curves in the spine. Pilates can help you to achieve better posture and restore the healthy spinal curves. For good alignment, there should be a long, shallow curve in the lower back (the "lordosis"). If your back arches too far from the mat, try padding under the tail of your spine with a folded towel.

If your back flattens into the mat, try placing a small rolled towel under your lower back so your spine curves gently away from the mat. Now check the position of your head—you may need to pad either under the neck or the back of your head to get a similarly gentle neck curve.

To check your standing posture, look front—and side-on in a mirror. Ideally, you should be symmetrical in the shoulders, rib cage, hips, knees, and ankles from the front, and the gentle curves should be visible from the side. Few of us have ideal posture, and it is best to think of it as a long-term aim that you can use Pilates to work toward. It is beyond the scope of this book to attempt individual correction—seek advice if you have problems related to your posture. Then use these exercises to help you work on improving posture with help from your Pilates teacher.

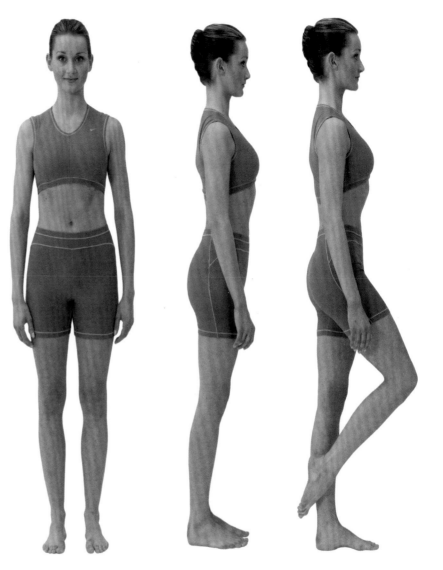

LOOKING in a mirror, the body should be symmetrical, limbs held evenly when at rest, and joints level.

SIDE VIEW The spine should form gentle S curves. Exaggerated or flattened curves reveal poor posture.

breathing

The most difficult part of Pilates is usually the breathing. For each exercise you have to align, center, breathe, and move. Your pattern of breathing should flow with the exercise. Original Pilates had set patterns of breathing for each move. Most teachers nowadays use breathing to help the effect of each exercise and improve control of posture and alignment.

You can practice Pilates breathing in the relaxation position (below). Place your hands on either side of your rib cage, and as you inhale, try to breathe gently into your hands—you should feel your back widen slightly. As you breathe out, press lightly with your palms so the ribs close a little

and roll down slightly toward the waist. This is the side breath or lateral breathing used in Pilates. It helps to offset the tendency to tense the neck and shoulders in shallow breathing or abdominal breathing (when the stomach pushes out and in with each breath), which make it harder to center and use the deep abdominals correctly.

Try to follow the breathing cues in the book, as they are designed to work with each exercise. Practically, you may want to grade your learning—begin with centering, alignment, and mentally rehearsing the moves, adding the breathing once you have mastered this.

THE RELAXATION position, with knees bent, spine relaxed, and hands on the pelvis, is the best position for practicing lateral breathing. This will help you achieve much more effective exercising in your Pilates routine.

WORK ON your posture in a sitting position. As in standing, look for a gentle curve in the spine and watch for tucking or overarching, which can indicate poor posture and alignment.

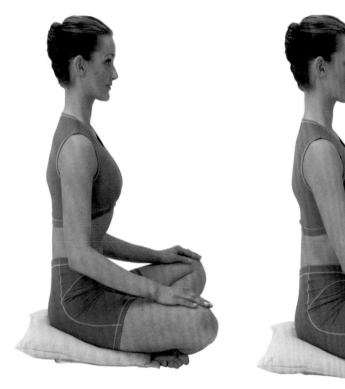

EXTEND your legs and check your posture again. Different positions put different stresses on the spine. Working from the center to support good spinal curves is the key to correct alignment.

TO CHECK whether you are breathing laterally, hold your hands on your ribs under your armpits. Lateral breathing should cause the ribs to move sideways into your hands.

BREATHING can be used to enhance stretches and change the focus of exercises. If you lie with your hands above your head, you can feel the upper back arch up as you breathe in and the chest expands.

flowing movement

The Pilates system was intended as flowing movement, not statically held postures. Watching someone who is experienced at Pilates perform the exercises, you will be struck by their economy of movement and their controlled, graceful execution.

The unique format of the photographs in this book will help you reproduce this, as you can see how one movement flows into the next. Have this in mind as you mentally rehearse your Pilates and as you are performing the exercises. You should be aiming for a steady, flowing movement between each stage of an exercise, as illustrated by the images.

Joseph Pilates believed that his innovative exercise method was the best way to achieve both health and happiness. This is the goal of Pilates, and as with any effective system, it should become part of your daily routine. It takes dedicated practice to master this thoughtful, mindful technique, but the benefits to mind and body, experienced by thousands of users already, will reward all your efforts. Refer to the information on the opposite page before starting to use the *Skills in Motion* Pilates sequences.

Suzanne Scott

USE SKILLS IN MOTION to achieve a flowing movement throughout your exercises. Each stage of every movement is pictured.

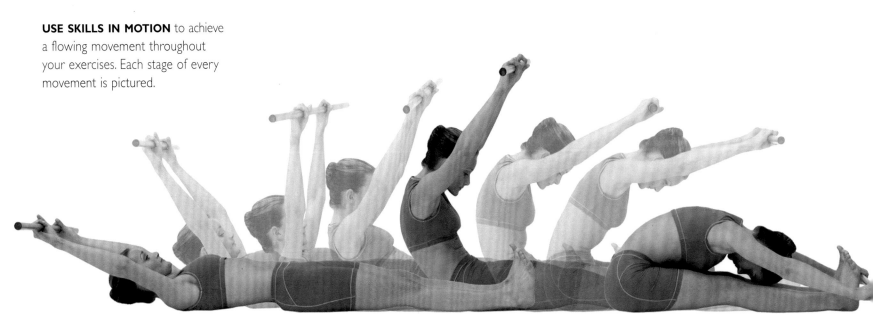

go with the flow

The special *Skills in Motion* images used in this book have been created to make sure that you see the whole of each exercise—not just selected highlights. Each exercise is labelled suitable for beginners, intermediate, or advanced students by a colored tab above the title. The captions along the bottom of the images provide additional information to help you perform the exercises confidently. Below this, another layer of information includes instructions for breathing and symbols indicating when to hold a position. The order the exercises are shown in the book is a suggested sequence only. Beginners should pick out suitable exercises, while intermediate and advanced exercisers can create their own program.

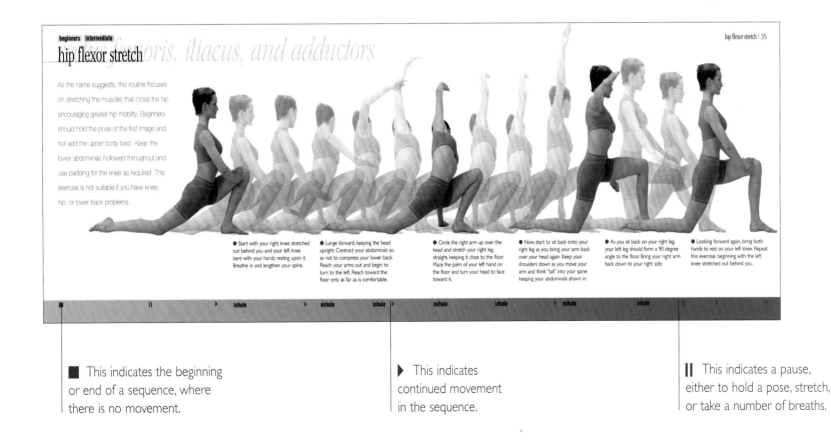

beginners intermediate

hip flexor stretch

...oris, iliacus, and adductors

hip flexor stretch | 35

As the name suggests, this routine focuses on stretching the muscles that cross the hip encouraging greater hip mobility. Beginners should hold the pose of the first image and not add the upper body twist. Keep the lower abdominals hollowed throughout and use padding for the knee as required. This exercise is not suitable if you have knee, hip, or lower back problems.

- Start with your right knee stretched out behind you and your left knee bent with your hands resting upon it. Breathe in and lengthen your spine.
- Lunge forward, keeping the head upright. Contract your abdominals so as not to compress your lower back. Reach your arms out and begin to turn to the left. Reach toward the floor only as far as is comfortable.
- Circle the right arm up over the head and stretch your right leg straight, keeping it close to the floor. Place the palm of your left hand on the floor and turn your head to face toward it.
- Now, start to sit back onto your right leg as you bring your arm back over your head again. Keep your shoulders down as you move your arm and think "tall" into your spine keeping your abdominals drawn in.
- As you sit back on your right leg, your left leg should form a 90 degree angle to the floor. Bring your right arm back down to your right side.
- Looking forward again, bring both hands to rest on your left knee. Repeat this exercise, beginning with the left knee stretched out behind you.

inhale   exhale   inhale   exhale   inhale   exhale   inhale

■ This indicates the beginning or end of a sequence, where there is no movement.

▶ This indicates continued movement in the sequence.

❚❚ This indicates a pause, either to hold a pose, stretch, or take a number of breaths.

turn outs *core stability and adductor stretch*

This is an excellent exercise to help increase flexibility in the hip joint by stretching your adductors.

As it is such a gentle exercise, it can be practiced by those with limited flexibility and those who are

new to Pilates. Focus on keeping the supporting leg still to challenge your core control.

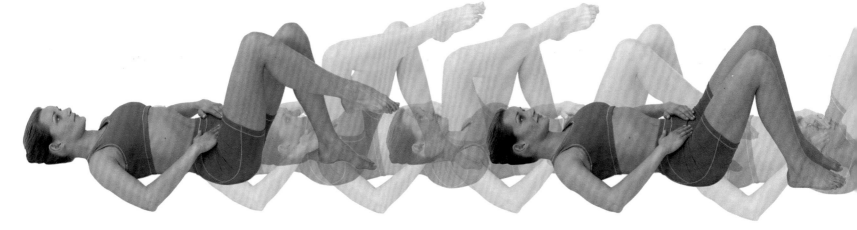

● Lie on your back with your knees bent and your hands on your pelvis. Breathe in and lengthen the spine.

● Bring your right leg up to a 90 degree angle with the knee still bent. Then turn out the knee. Keep your back flat on the floor and your neck relaxed.

● Point your foot as you turn the knee. You should feel the stretch on your inner thigh.

● Bring the knee back down again and rest for a few moments with your hands on your pelvis. Keep your neck lengthened and your gaze toward the sky.

| | ❚❚ begin to exhale | ▶ exhale | ▶ inhale | ▶ |

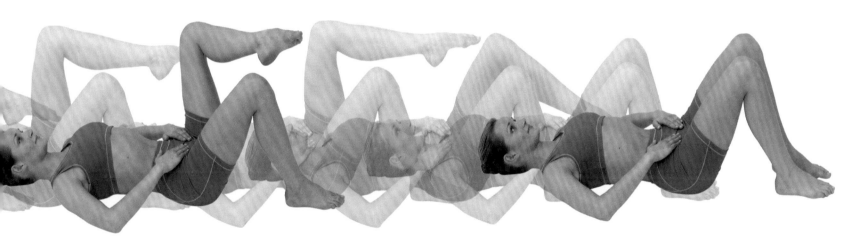

Then, raise your left leg up, pointing the toes as you do so, and keeping the supporting leg still and steady. Keep your shoulders down and relaxed.

● Raise the leg up to a 90 degree angle and vthen turn the knee out as before. Again, make sure your lower back remains on the floor as you perform this stretch.

● Bring your left leg down to the floor again. Make sure you keep the movement slow, controlled, and precise.

● Finish this exercise in the same position as you started. Relax your whole body and breathe deeply.

sliding arms and legs *houlder girdle stability*

This exercise helps to develop your "center." You should focus on keeping your pelvis and ribs still as your arms and legs work. Aim for flowing movements of your limbs as your abdominals draw in to support your spine and create your center.

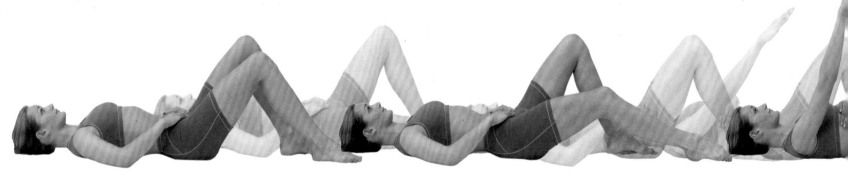

● Start by lying on your back with your knees bent and your feet flat on the floor. Have your arms relaxed and resting on your stomach. Breathe in and lengthen the spine.

● Start to lower your right leg down toward the floor, keeping your left leg bent and your shoulders relaxed.

● Make sure your neck is lengthened and not tense. Slide the leg down to the floor without locking your knee. Flex, point, and slide it back up again. Repeat using the left leg.

● Put your left hand onto your right rib. Raise your right arm in the air. Point your fingers away from you and concentrate on isolating the movement in the arm so as to avoid hunching the shoulder.

inhale ▶ exhale inhale ▶ begin to exhale ▶

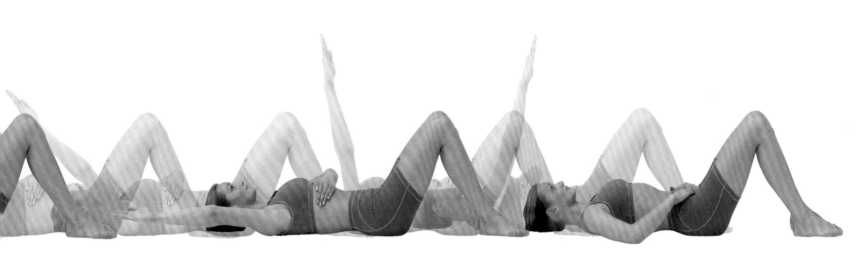

● Bring your right arm back toward the floor. Keep your arm lengthened and make sure this is a slow and controlled movement.

● Extend your arm right over your head so it is aligned with the rest of your body. Keep your back flat on the floor and be careful not to let your neck become tense. Breathe in. Do not force your arm back.

● Bring the arm back down again toward your legs and rest it on your hip. Repeat this arm movement with your left arm.

● Finish the exercise in the starting position. Have both hands resting on your hips and your body relaxed and aligned.

exhale   ▶ **inhale**   **exhale**   ‖   ▶   ‖

knee and leg circles *core stability and hip rotators*

This original Pilates exercise improves the pelvic stability and the mobility of the hip joint. Beginners should keep both legs bent at the knee throughout and use the stretch band for support. The leg circles demand a high level of core control and flexibility. Do not attempt them if you are a beginner. If you have lower back problems, seek medical advice before using any part of this exercise.

- Lie on your back with your knees bent and your arms by your side. Breathe in and lengthen the spine. Pick up your stretch band and place it under your left knee.

- Allow your leg to relax and drop slightly to the side. Don't move your legs, let the movement come from your hips. This loosens your hips and teaches you to move from the hip. Repeat with the other leg.

- Return your knees to the center and put the stretch band to one side. Have your arms by your side with the palms facing down. Raise your left leg up in the air and extend it as you reach.

- Now, draw some wide semicircles in the air with your toes pointed. Remember to avoid arching your back and keep your neck relaxed.

‖ exhale ▶ inhale exhale ▶ exhale ▶

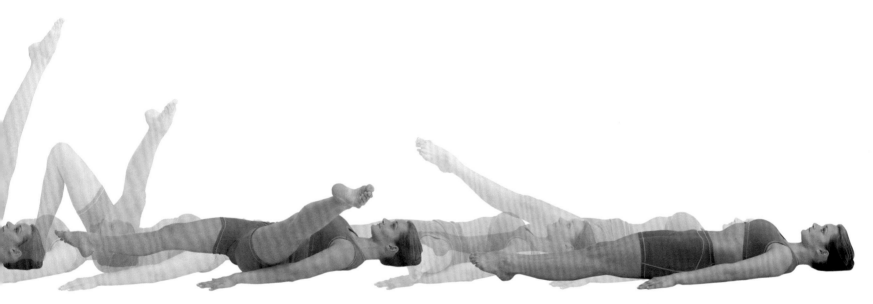

● Stretch the right leg out with
he toes pointed. Keep it raised 1–2
nches (2–4 centimeters) above the
oor and perform another semicircle
 this position.

● Try to make the semicircle as wide
as possible. However, do not force or
strain your legs in any way. Keep your
back flat on the floor and the rest of
your body still.

● As you complete the semicircle
concentrate on keeping your legs
lengthened, but don't lock your knees.

● When you have finished this
exercise, lower both legs to the floor,
and then repeat the whole routine
with your right leg.

first connection

arm reach and biceps curl

Latissimus dorsi, biceps, and deltoids

This exercise works the major muscles of the upper back and arms. If you focus on the position of your shoulders (don't hunch or pinch the shoulder blades together), it will help to develop stability in your shoulder girdle. Intermediate exercisers can use weights to add resistance.

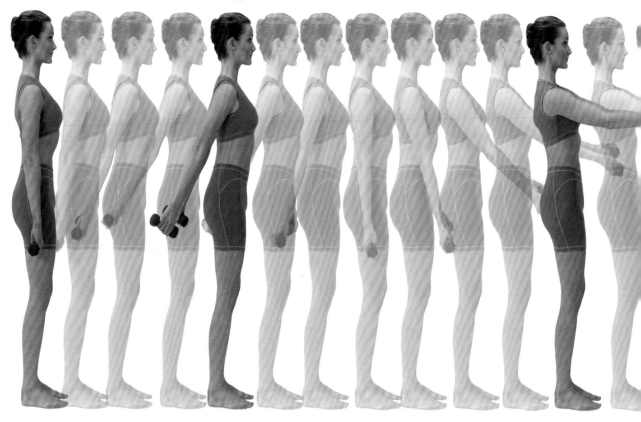

● Begin the exercise in the standing position with your hands by your side. Keep your back lengthened and be careful not to arch it at any point in the stretch. Keep your shoulders relaxed and wide.

● Before beginning the exercise, breathe in, contract your abdominals, and lengthen the spine. Grip the weights securely with your palms facing back. Squeeze your arms into your body and feel the biceps relax.

● Breathe out as you move your arms slowly back. Concentrate on lengthening your arms as they move backward, as though you were reaching into the floor. Keep your elbows soft, your shoulders relaxed.

● As you begin to turn your hands around to come forward, take a breath in. Keep your eyes horizontal and focus on a spot directly ahead of you. Concentrate on keeping the back of the neck long and the head upright

▶ **inhale** ▶ **exhale** ▶ **inhale** ▶

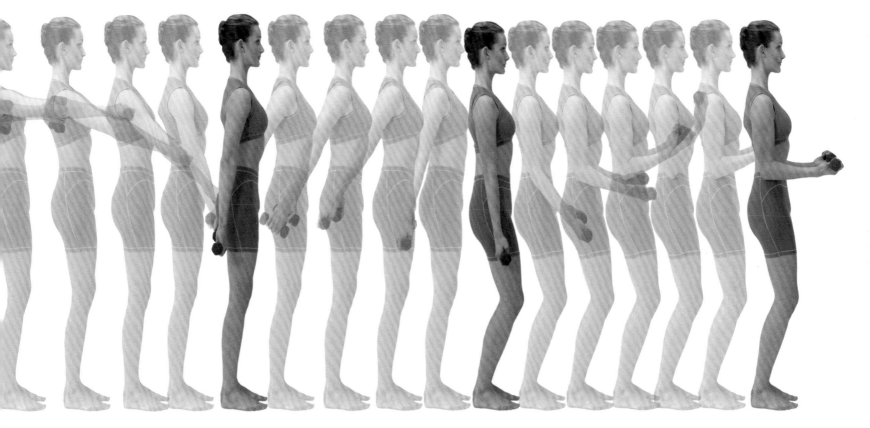

Breathe out as the arms are extended all the way forward with your palms upright. Keep your spine straight and imagine that the tail of it is rooted into the ground.

● As you breathe in, begin to turn your hands around to face the ground and start to take your arms back to your sides again. Be careful not to let your weight move back. Breathe out as your arms go all the way back.

● Once the arms are back, take a deep breath in, then on the out breath, bring your arms forward again, bending your knees as you do. Bring your arms back to the side of your body.

● Now curl the forearms up, keeping the upper arms very still. As you raise your hands, keep your wrists straight and do not allow your elbows to drop. Breathe in as you release the arms and then relax.

exhale ▶ inhale ▶ exhale ▶ inhale ▶ exhale ▶ ‖ inhale ▶ ▐▐▐

chest stretch

pectorals arm rotators and deltoids

This exercise strengthens the major muscles of the arms, shoulders, and upper back. Beginners should perform this without weights. People with shoulder problems should avoid the arm raise and only take the "offering" as far as is comfortable. Keep your head, neck, and shoulders aligned.

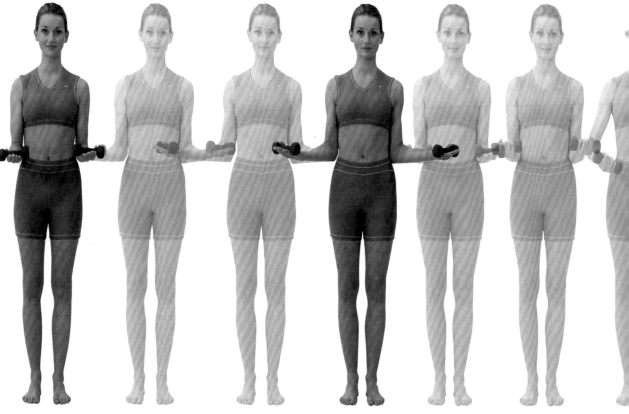

● Start with the arms bent at the elbows, holding the weights in the palms of the hand with the fingers pointing forward. Grip the weights with your thumbs. If you are not using weights, use the same hand position.

● Breathe in to prepare, checking that the spine is lengthened and the shoulders wide and relaxed. Start the chest stretch by moving the hands out from the body, keeping the elbows locked at your waist.

● Continue the stretch as far as you can—the ideal is for both lower arms to end up in a straight line with each other. Move the hands back to the center and then repeat the stretch four times.

● Now grip the weights and start to lower your arms, bending the elbows out as you go.

▶ inhale   exhale   ▶   inhale

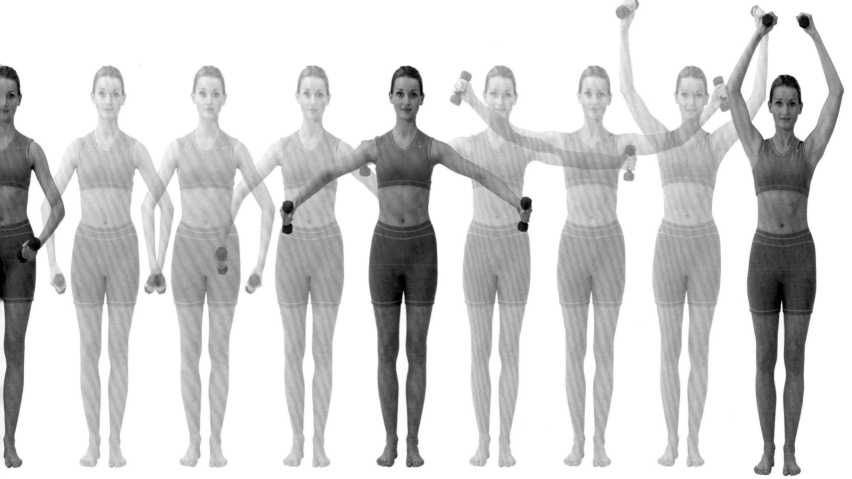

When the weights are level with our pelvis, hold the position for a econd and take a breath. Again, check hat your spine is still lengthened and our shoulders are not hunched.

● As you breathe out, start to lift your arms up and out to the sides. As the hands rise, begin to turn them so the palms are facing forward.

● When your arms reach shoulder level, your palms should be facing forward. As you continue to reach up, keep rotating the hands until the palms are uppermost.

● Steadily bring the arms together above your head. They shouldn't touch, but should rest about fist width apart. Breathe in as you let your arms return to your sides. Repeat the arm raise four times.

roll down against wall and sit back extensors and core stability

This is a classic Pilates exercise, often used at the beginning or end of a class. It helps relieve muscle tension in your neck and shoulders, and improves the flexibility of your spine. Keep your hips over your knees as you roll—do not allow the pelvis to twist. bent throughout. You should not attempt this exercise if you have lower back problems.

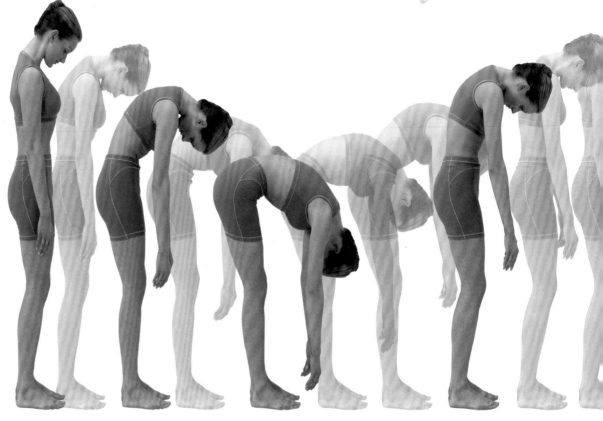

● Start in the standing position with your feet apart and your knees relaxed. Breathe in and lengthen your spine. Pull in your abdominal muscles and gently lower your neck forward.

● Breathe out as you let your arms fall forward and your back curve. Relax your head and shoulders, and pay attention to your spine as it gently relaxes, curling over. Keep the movement gentle and controlled.

● Breathe in and start to roll slowly back up to the standing position. Imagine a string is attached to the crown of your head, pulling your body up in a straight line.

‖ inhale ▶ exhale ▶ inhale ▶

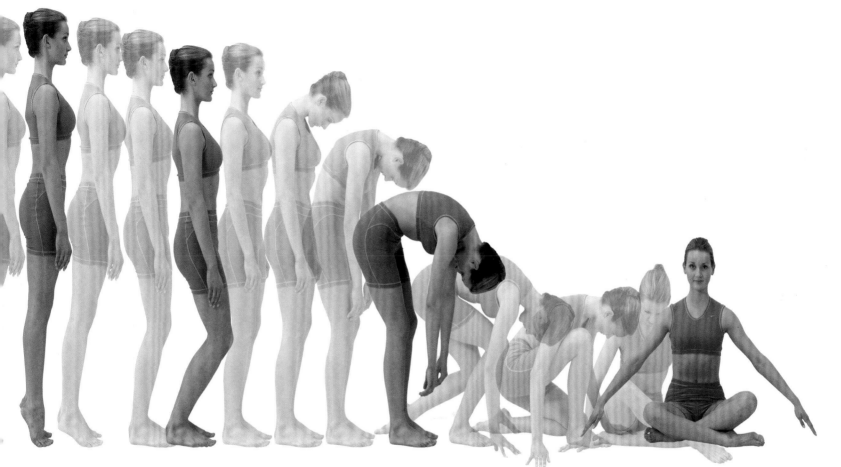

Stand up straight and then stand tall the tips of your feet. Imagine that ou are leaning against a wall so your ottom doesn't push back or sway rward.

● Come back down so your feet are flat. Bend your knees and straighten them again. Then, breathe in and contract your abdominals as you prepare to start rolling your head, neck, and back forward, as before.

● Bend your knees again, place your fingers on the floor for support, and kneel down. Put one leg back as you prepare to sit on the floor.

● Sit down in the cross-legged position and extend your arms at each side of your body. Lengthen your spine and neck, and relax.

neck and shoulder stretch *mid and upper back extensors*

This exercise stretches the entire spine forward (into flexion). It is not suitable for those with neck and lower back problems, but can otherwise be used to release muscle tension. Try to keep your lower abdominals drawn in to support your spine and use your breathing to relax into the stretch.

● Begin the exercise cross-legged, with your spine upright and your arms out to the sides, fingertips pointing to the floor. Breathe in and lengthen the spine, keeping your lower abdominals contracted.

● Lean your head to the right and start to lift your right hand. Keep the left arm in position and the shoulders relaxed. Straighten the head again at this point.

● Continue to raise the hand, focusing on keeping the spine lengthened and the shoulders loose and soft.

● As the hand rises above horizontal start to turn the palm in toward your head. At the same time, turn to face the hand as the arm hooks over.

inhale ▶	begin to exhale ▶	exhale ▶ inhale

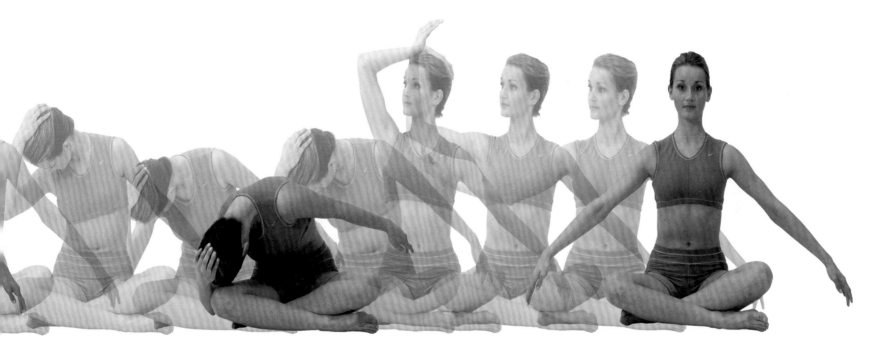

Lightly hold the crown of your head. Take a breath here but do not pull on the neck, allowing the weight of the head to come forward for a gentle stretch.

● Breathe out as you bend from the neck. Let the spine gently roll down, using your hand for support. Continue the stretch as far as you can comfortably go. Breathe in and out again to deepen the stretch.

● When you have bent fully forward from the waist, take four breaths in the lowered position. Then, start to sit up again. Keep your hand on your head all the way up and don't release until you are upright.

● Return to the center position. Relax, lengthen the spine, and relax the shoulders. Now repeat the entire stretch on the other side.

exhale ▶   ‖ inhale and exhale x 4 ▶ inhale ▶   exhale

leg, spine, and hip stretch

back extensors and hip rotators

This advanced sequence develops flexibility in the back and hips in preparation for advanced exercises. Do not attempt it if you have neck, hip, or lower back problems. Beginners should keep the knees bent. Do not use the open leg stretch unless you are an advanced exerciser.

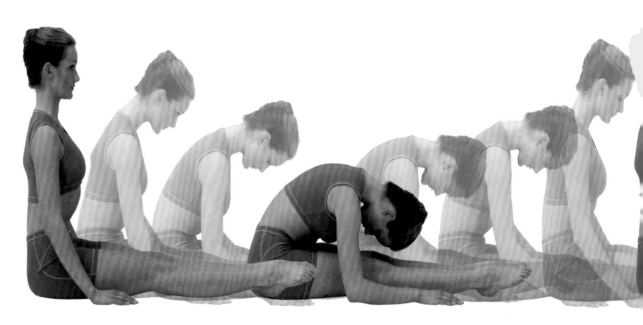

● It is important to prepare properly for this exercise. Breathe in, lengthen the spine, and loosen the shoulders. Relax your hips and sit into your pelvis. Beginners should sit on a cushion or low box.

● Keep your hands flat on the floor as you slide them forward. Move down from your neck, letting your spine curl gently and keeping your abdominals pulled into your spine.

● You will feel tension all along the spine, as well as in the legs and buttocks. Continue the stretch as far as you can, but don't force yourself beyond your limits. Take six breaths at the farthest point of the stretch.

● Gently roll back up from your waist, stacking up the middle of the spine and finally the neck. Keep your lower abdominals contracted.

▶ inhale   exhale   ‖ inhale and exhale x 6   ▶ inhale   ▶

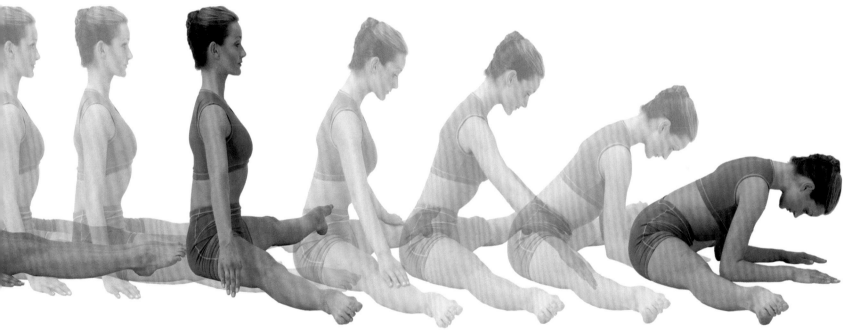

● Take a few seconds to make sure the spine is lengthened, the pelvis neutral, and the shoulders relaxed. Now, start to bring your legs out to the sides, keeping them straight. Beginners should not attempt this.

● Bring the arms forward over the legs and point the fingers in front of you at the floor.

● Start bending forward from the waist, letting your lower arms take your weight. Flatten the palms on the floor and keep them in place, bending at the elbows as the back lowers.

● Keep your abdominals drawn in. Do not force your hips or the forward bend of the spine. You should aim for a comfortable stretch.

hip reach *and hip rotators and adductors*

This advanced exercise takes Pilates principles and applies them to a challenging stretch sequence. The focus of the stretch should be right at the fingertips with the rest of your arm and spine flowing behind. Aim for grace and flowing coordination. You should not attempt this exercise if you are a beginner or you suffer from lower back or hip problems.

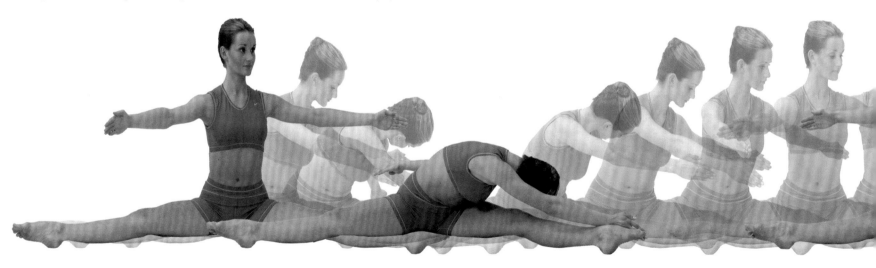

● Stretch your legs out as far as possible and raise your arms up level with your shoulders, palms forward. Relax the shoulders, zip up, and make sure the pelvis is neutral. Start to twist to the left from the waist.

● As you twist, the arms should stay in line with each other. The whole of your upper body is pivoting from the waist, challenging hip muscles such as the obliques and the muscles of the lower back and upper leg.

● As you come over the left leg, twist your head to face behind you. Try to touch your toes. Use your breathing to enhance the stretch (lowering on the out breath). Keep the lower abdominals contracted.

● Now rise from the waist again. Bring your arms back in line with each other as your back straightens up. Keep your lower abdominals hollow as you stack up your spine.

| ■ | ▶ | inhale | exhale | ▶ | inhale | exhale | ▶ | inhale | ▶ |

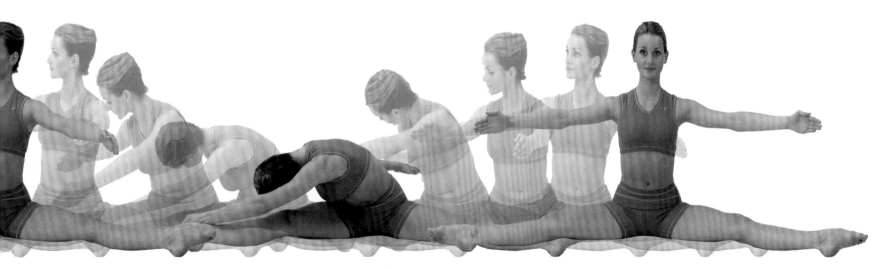

Don't rest in the center position, move straight on to stretch on the other side. Twist from your waist to the right, keeping the arms in line with each other. Remember to keep focusing on your abdominals.

● As the head comes forward over the leg, turn it to face behind you. Reach your left hand to try to touch your toes. Extend the stretch as far as you can without forcing yourself beyond your natural range.

● Come back up to the center, untwisting and rising from the waist. Keep the arms outstretched and your fingers and toes pointed. Keep your lower abdominals drawn in to support your spine with each movement.

● Once back at the center, bring the legs together and the arms down to finish the exercise.

exhale ▶ inhale ▶ exhale ▶

hip flexor stretch *oris, iliacus, and adductors*

As the name suggests, this routine focuses on stretching the muscles that cross the hip encouraging greater hip mobility. Beginners should hold the pose of the first image and not add the upper body twist. Keep the lower abdominals hollowed throughout and use padding for the knee as required. This exercise is not suitable if you have knee, hip, or lower back problems.

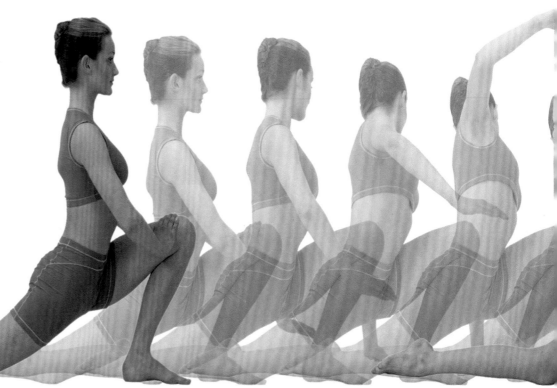

● Start with your right knee stretched out behind you and your left knee bent with your hands resting upon it. Breathe in and lengthen your spine.

● Lunge forward, keeping the head upright. Contract your abdominals so as not to compress your lower back. Reach your arms out and begin to turn to the left. Reach toward the floor only as far as is comfortable.

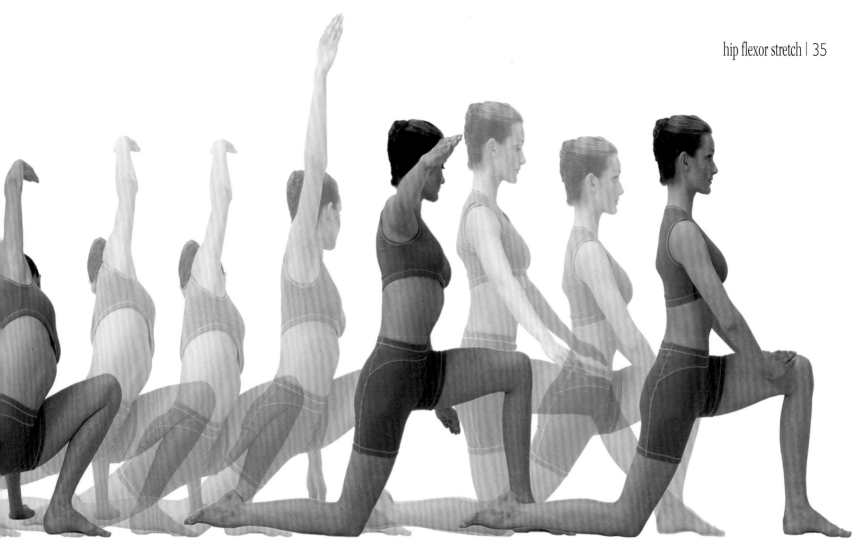

● Circle the right arm up over the
[h]ead and stretch your right leg
[s]traight, keeping it close to the floor.
[P]lace the palm of your left hand on
[th]e floor and turn your head to face
[t]oward it.

● Now, start to sit back onto your
right leg as you bring your arm back
over your head again. Keep your
shoulders down as you move your
arm and think "tall" into your spine
keeping your abdominals drawn in.

● As you sit back on your right leg,
your left leg should form a 90 degree
angle to the floor. Bring your right arm
back down to your right side.

● Looking forward again, bring both
hands to rest on your left knee. Repeat
this exercise, beginning with the left
knee stretched out behind you.

curl, twist, and airplane

oblique abdominals and hip flexors

This exercise is a demanding workout for the whole abdominal group of muscles (especially the external and internal obliques). Beginners should build strength by practicing the simple rolling back action at the start of the sequence, progressing through arms bent to the full version shown at the end. Do not attempt this exercise if you have lower back problems.

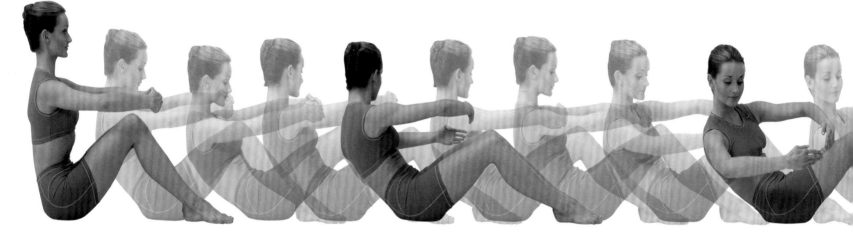

● Sit upright with your knees bent and your feet flat on the floor. If this is uncomfortable, sit on a cushion. Have your arms rounded in front of you and above your knees. Breathe in and contract your lower abdominals.

● Breathe out and gradually roll back, lowering your back only as far as you can maintain good abdominal control.

● Turn your body to the left in mid "sit back." Release the tension between your shoulders and engage the stomach muscles to keep your back supported. Move your arms and head together as you turn to the left.

● Then, come back to the center and twist to the right. Use your lower abdominals to keep the pose smooth. Return to the center and repeat this movement on both sides three times.

■ inhale   ‖ exhale   ▶ exhale   ▶ inhale   exhale

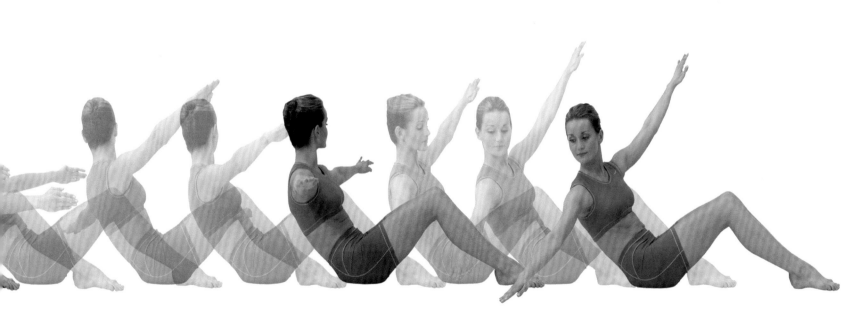

● After these repetitions, return to the center. Keep leaning back and begin to open your arms out to the sides. Twist to the left, putting the left hand down on the floor and the right hand parallel pointing up.

● Keep the arms straight and stretched and come back to the horizontal position. Remember to keep your shoulders soft and relaxed all the time.

● Now, twist to the right, turning your head toward your right hand and raising your left arm into the air as you turn. Keep your buttocks firmly on the floor and concentrate on making this a controlled, slow movement.

● Reach your right hand down to the floor and feel the work in your oblique muscles. Repeat this airplane exercise on both sides.

upper ab curl *abdominal muscles*

This exercise works all four muscles of the abdominal group (rectus abdominis, internal and external obliques, and transversus). The transversus abdominis, responsible for abdominal hollowing, should be gently drawn in toward your spine before you begin to curl. This is what turns a generic sit-up into a powerful Pilates move. Try to keep your pelvis steady and your lower back neutral.

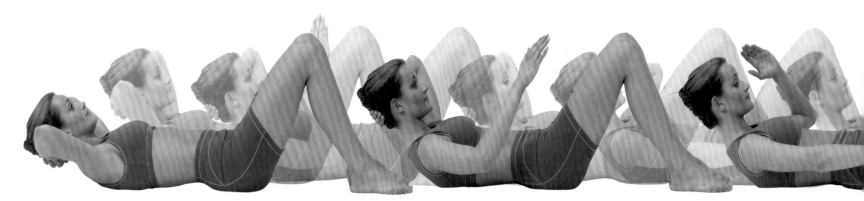

● Start this exercise lying on the floor with your knees bent. Have your arms behind your head to support your neck. Breathe in and lengthen the spine.

● Lift the head and shoulders off the floor. Curl up one vertebra at a time to a comfortable position. Scoop your stomach muscles in to support your lower back and keep your pelvis in the neutral position.

● Bring your right hand forward toward your hip. Keep the other arm behind your head to make sure your head is in the correct position. Lengthen and relax your neck. Fix your gaze slightly above your knees.

● Extend your right arm so it is level with your hip. Then start to bring the other arm down, making sure you keep your neck in the same position. Beginners can support the head throughout swopping hands.

▌▌ exhale   ▶   inhale   ▶   exhale   ▶

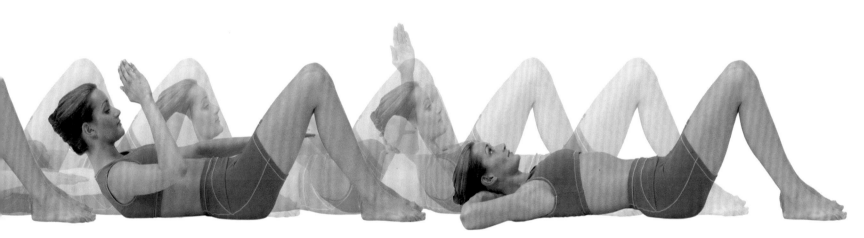

As you extend your left arm down toward your hip, start to bring the right arm up toward your head again.

● After you have stretched your left arm forward, start to bring it back toward your neck again. Keep your spine in neutral and your lower abdominals drawn in.

● Then put both hands behind your neck and roll back down on the floor to relax.

● This exercise can be repeated as many times as you like, but you must be careful not to strain your neck and shoulders as you perform it.

hale ▶ **begin to exhale** **exhale** ‖ ▶ ‖

crisscross

oblique abdominals and hip flexors

This original Pilates exercise is excellent for strengthening the abdominals and training upper and lower body coordination. Beginners can start by rotating the upper body only and keeping both feet on the floor. Progress to holding the feet in the air and then gradually begin to straighten them as your strength improves. Do not attempt this exercise if you have neck and lower back problems.

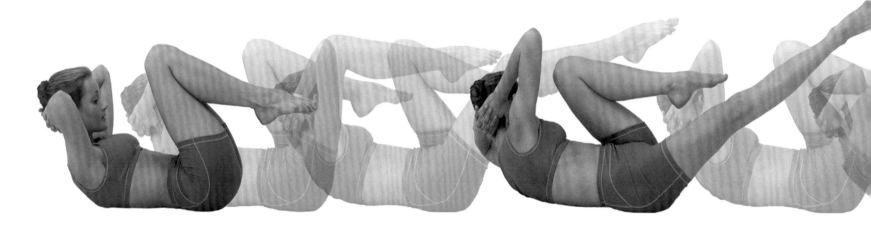

● Lie on your back with your hands behind your head. Contract your lower abdominals then lift your head and bend your knees into your chest. Keep your elbows extended as much as possible.

● Start to extend you right leg out; as you do so, begin to twist your upper body so your right elbow is aiming for your left knee. Keep hollowing the lower abdominals and allow the lower back to flatten slightly.

● Make sure you are lifting from below your shoulder in order to reach the knee and not twisting from the shoulder socket. Bring the elbow so it almost touches the left knee. Hold the position and breathe out.

● As you start to move the right leg back, begin to extend the opposite leg out in front of you.

■ ‖ inhale ▶ exhale ▶ inhale ▶

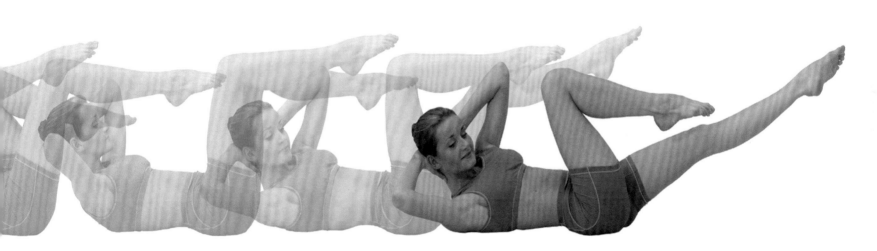

● Aim your left elbow for your right knee, but imagine that your center is anchored to the floor so you don't rock your body from hip to hip.

● As you extend your left leg, do not allow it to drop too low in front of you. You can maintain control of the leg position by squeezing your buttocks and doing the exercise slowly.

● Concentrate on lifting and twisting from your waist. You should feel the work above and below your waistline.

● When the left leg is fully extended, hold the stretch and exhale completely. Complete up to 10 times, then pull your knees into your chest to relax back on the floor.

exhale ▶ exhale inhale ▶ exhale ⏸

waist twists

quadratus lumborum

This exercise works the oblique abdominals and stretches a major side flexor of the spine and the spinal rotators. It also increases the mobility of the spine especially in the thoracic area. Beginners or those who have had back problems should keep their feet on the floor and only attempt the version shown in the first four images. Do not attempt this exercise if you have current back problems.

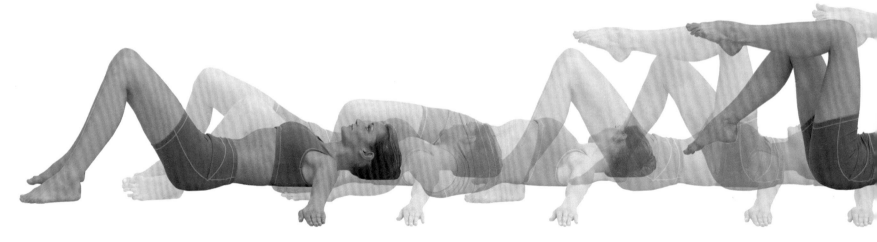

● Start the exercise by lying on your back with your feet flat on the floor and your knees bent. Breathe in deeply and lengthen the spine.

● Stretch your arms out to the side so they are parallel with your shoulders. Pause.

● As you breathe out, drop your knees comfortably to your left side while turning your head in the other direction. Use your breathing to increase the stretch and keep your lower abdominals contracted.

● Return your legs to the center and then repeat the exercise on the other side, dropping your knees to the right and turning your head to the left.

inhale   ❚❚   ▶   exhale   ▶   inhale   ▶

For an advanced level of Pilates, begin this exercise with your knees in the air at right angles to your body. Place a tennis ball between your knees and grip it.

● Then, twist to the left with your legs, keeping the ball in the same position, and turn your head to the right.

● Return your legs to the starting position and then repeat on the other side. Concentrate on lengthening the spine and neck as you do this exercise, and make sure you twist from the waist and not the shoulders.

● Inhaling, refill your lungs, feel your chest expand as you return to the center and relax.

creating energy

hip lift
oblique abdominals and glutes

The principal challenge here is to keep your body balanced and steady while the leg is elevated.

You will feel your pelvis tip to the side or sway as each leg comes up. Try to keep your pelvis and

spine aligned by using your hands at your side. Beginners should practice just raising the heel

before progressing to straightening the leg. Do not attempt this exercise if you have back problems.

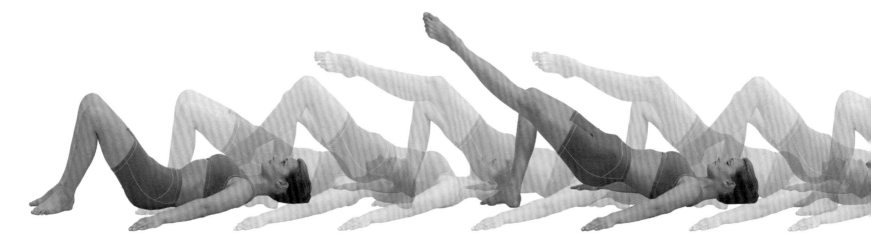

● Begin the exercise in the relaxation position, with the feet flat on the floor and the knees bent. Beginners should aim to lift the heel only at first, before progressing to lifting the leg.

● On an out breath, pull in the lower abdominals and start to lift the pelvis up to wherever is comfortable. Now start to lift the left foot off the ground.

● Continue reaching up with the left leg until it is pointing about 40 degrees from the floor. Pause here for a second and breathe in.

● As you breathe out, contract your lower abdominals and lower the left leg to the floor again. When it reaches the floor, pause again and breathe in.

| ■ | inhale | ▶ | exhale | | | inhale | ‖ | exhale | ▶ | inhale |

Now, repeat the sequence with the right leg. Remember to lift the leg on an outbreath and pause when you reach the straight leg position.

● Breathe in as you hold the position. Feel the leg lengthening at the knee, pulling away from the hips, which remain steady and square.

● Breathe out as you lower the right leg to the floor. Do this with control; don't just let it collapse.

● With both feet grounded, bring the pelvis back to the floor. As with the feet, don't let the pelvis collapse. Lower it slowly and gently, keeping the lower abdominals hollowed.

tree climb

hamstrings and gastrocnemius

This is an advanced hamstring and calf stretch performed in lying and sitting positions. It requires good abdominal control to keep the pelvis steady. Beginners may attempt a modified version by keeping the knees bent in both parts of the exercise. Always contract the lower abdominals to support the back. Do not attempt this exercise if you have lower back problems.

● Begin the sequence lying flat on the floor with your arms by your sides and your palms facing down. Inhale and lengthen the spine.

● Contract your lower abdominals as you lift your right knee. Lift both arms toward your raised knee. Bring your knee back to 90 degrees to the body, and place your hands on the front of the knee, flexing your foot to point.

● Pull the knee back into the chest and take the hands onto the inside of the thigh, just below the knee. Keep drawing in your lower abdominals as you straighten your raised leg to a comfortable vertical position.

● Carefully straighten the extended leg, bringing it in toward your body. Flex the heel so you feel a stretch—not a strain—in the hamstrings and calf muscles. You should not feel anything in the back.

| inhale | exhale | ▶ | inhale | ▶ | breathe normally |

Now lift your head and shoulders from the floor toward your raised leg. As you do so, slowly move your hands to your leg to avoid straining your neck and shoulders. Keep your lower abdominals pulled in to your spine and make sure your pelvis is level.

● Continue raising your body and moving your hands up your leg until they are gripping the calf muscles just below the ankle. Both legs should be straight with toes pointed. Inhale deeply and hold the pose. Keep the abdominals engaged and pelvis square.

● Now, release the stretch and walk your hands back down the leg as you slowly lower your back toward the floor. Once your hands are on the back of your thigh again, bend your leg and bring the foot down to rest flat on the floor.

● Extend your leg once it is back on the floor, making sure both toes point away from the body. Bring your arms down to your sides with palms facing the floor. Relax and breathe deeply, then repeat the exercise with the other leg.

xhale   inhale || exhale   inhale   ▶   breathe normally ||

adductor stretch *and hip rotators*

This exercise stretches the inner thigh. To maintain good pelvic alignment, you will need to coordinate the deep hip and abdominal muscles. Aim for a gentle stretch in the inner thighs—do not push or force the legs, and don't arch the back. Beginners should perform the stretch by keeping both feet on the floor, allowing the knees to drop out while keeping the pelvis steady. At intermediate level, the knees should be kept bent throughout. The straight leg version shown is highly advanced. Do not attempt this exercise if you have lower back, hip, or knee problems.

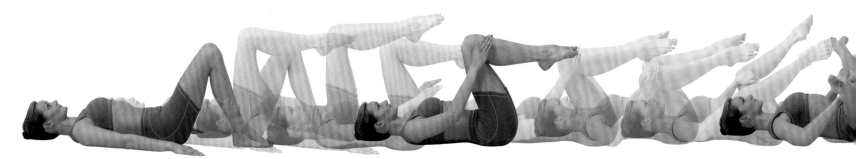

● Lie on your back with your knees bent and your feet flat on the floor. Take a deep breath in and lengthen the spine.

● Lift your right leg up so it is at a 90 degree angle to your body. Then, bring your left leg up so it is parallel to it. Keep your abdominals drawn in and your pelvis steady.

● Grip your knees with your hands and start to open your legs as far apart as you can. Activate the abs to avoid arching your back off the floor as you do this. Keep your neck lengthened and relaxed.

● Change the grip to the inside of your thighs and extend your legs out straight as far as you find comfortable. There should be no pain in your knees. Point your toes out. Hold this position for a few breaths.

Ⅱ inhale ▶ **begin to exhale** ▶ **exhale** ▶

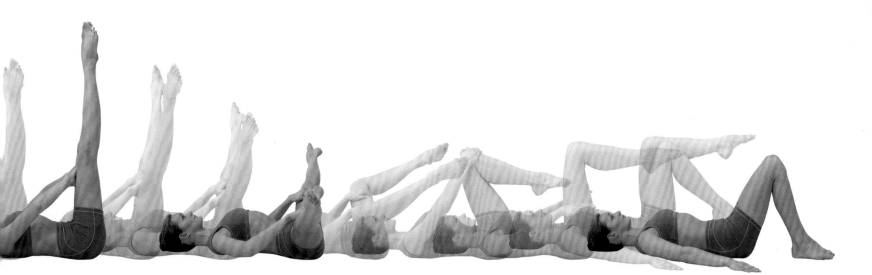

Then, close your legs, keeping them
raight so they are at a 90 degree
ngle to your body. Keep your toes
ointed and your back firmly on the
oor. Breathe in.

● Lower your legs back down again,
keeping your abdominals pulled in to
your spine as you do. Remember, this
is a highly advanced stretch, you
should not push into discomfort.

● Bend your knees from this position
and grip the outside of your knees to
pull them up to the center again. Then
put both of your arms on the floor,
parallel to your body with your palms
facing down.

● Lower the right leg to the floor and
then the left leg. Take a deep breath in
and then out. Relax.

leg switch

abdominals and hip flexors

Although the focus of movement in this exercise is the legs, the hard work takes place in the abdominal muscles, which need to be activated to support the spine. Gently press your spine into the floor without tucking your pelvis under. Don't arch the lower back and avoid this exercise if you have neck or lower back problems.

- Start in the relaxation position, with the feet flat and the knees bent. Place your hands behind your head. Breathe in as you prepare, and contract your lower abdominals to gently flatten the spine into the floor.

- Breathe out as you lift one and then the other leg up so the lower leg is horizontal. Now, take your legs up to the vertical.

- Breathe in at the vertical position, then breathe out as you lift your head and shoulders up off the floor. Keep your abdominals engaged and your pelvis steady.

- Keeping your head raised, lower your left leg. Keep your spine straight and don't let your back arch or your shoulder blades come off the floor. Lower your leg only as far as you can keep your abdominals pulling in.

| inhale | exhale | inhale | exhale | inhale | exhale |

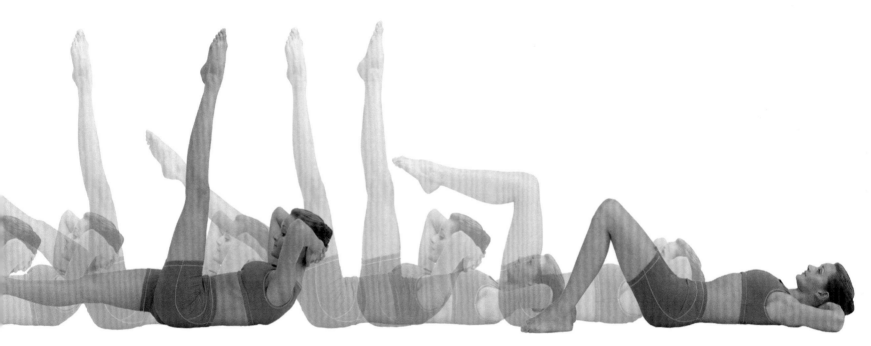

Bring the left leg back to join the right leg. Now allow the right leg to lower to the floor. Do not allow your pelvis to roll or twist.

● Keep the toes pointed out as your right leg reaches horizontal. The leg shouldn't actually touch the floor at the horizontal level.

● Now bring the right leg back up to the vertical and bend at the knees to bring both legs to a 90 degree angle.

● Continue to breathe out as you lower your feet to the floor and relax the pelvis and the spine.

arm switch and triceps curls

pectorals, deltoids, and triceps

This exercise challenges the stability of the ribcage and shoulder girdle. Focus on keeping your spine aligned on the floor. Don't let your back arch or your ribs flare as your arms go over your head. If you feel any strain, make the movements smaller. Do not perform this exercise if you have shoulder problems. For the tricep curl, focus on the elbow joint, keeping the upper arm still.

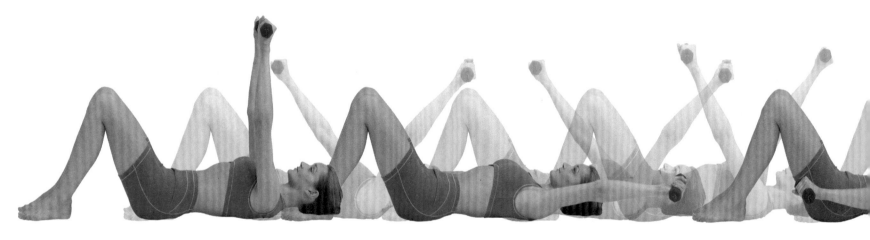

● Begin in the relaxation position with your arms vertical. Keep your elbows soft—don't lock them. Breathe in as you prepare to move your arms.

● Breathe out as you lower both arms straight down in parallel with your body. The left arm goes back behind your head, the right comes down beside your waist. Keep the wrists in line with the rest of the arms.

● Breathe in as you aim to take the arm to the horizontal, without letting it touch the floor. Breathe out and contract your abdominals as you start to raise your arms back to the vertical.

● As your arms come together, take a breath, and concentrate on correcting your posture—lengthen the spine, loosen the elbows, and soften the shoulders. Now breathe out as you begin to lower your arms again.

■ ▶ **inhale**   **exhale**   ‖ **inhale** ▶ **exhale**   ‖ **inhale** ▶ **exhale**

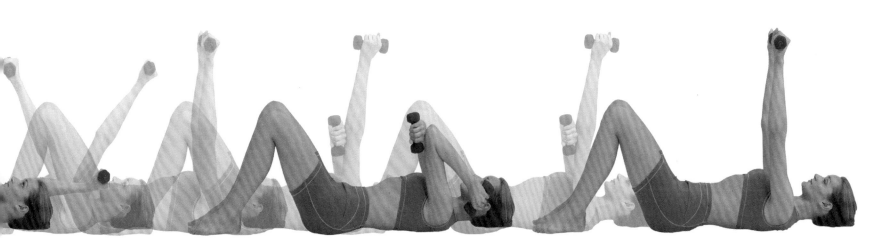

This time, lower each arm in the opposite direction. Again, try to keep the wrists straight, don't flare your ribs, and keep your spine lengthened.

● Breathe out as you lower your arms, breathe in when they reach the horizontal position, and then breathe out as you raise them back to vertical. Repeat this exercise eight times.

● Now, place your right hand behind your left elbow to support it for the tricep curl. The tricep is the muscle on the back of the upper arm. Slowly lift the weight back up to the vertical, pivoting around the elbow.

● Take the weight down to ear level and then raise it back up to vertical. Now, repeat with the other arm. Do up to eight sets of this exercise.

| II | inhale | ▶ | exhale | II | inhale | ▶ | exhale | inhale |

core dynamics

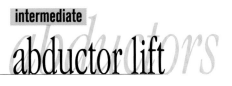

abductor lift

This exercise works the buttock muscles (gluteals), while the muscles along the back of your legs (hamstrings and gastrocnemius) are lengthening. It also challenges your core control in the shoulder girdle and pelvis as you work to keep your torso steady. Intermediate and advanced exercisers can use leg weights to add resistance. Beginners can attempt a less demanding version, keeping the working leg bent and the lift small. Do not attempt this if you have knee or lower back problems.

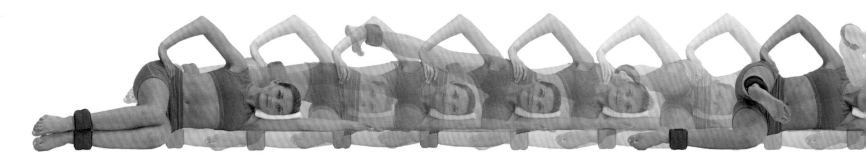

● Start on your left side, with your knees bent at a right angle to your body and your right hand on your hip. Have your head resting on a towel or small pillow, as this will help to keep your neck straight.

● Breathe in and begin to lift your right leg up. Breathe out and stretch your leg straight in line with your body. Keep your lower abs contracted.

● Now, flex the right foot and point the toes to the floor. Raise your leg a few inches and then lower it again. Repeat this up to four times, depending on strength and stamina.

● Pull your leg forward in front of you to hip level. Raise your leg up an inch from this position and then lower it.

■   ‖ inhale   exhale   inhale   ▶   exhale   ▶

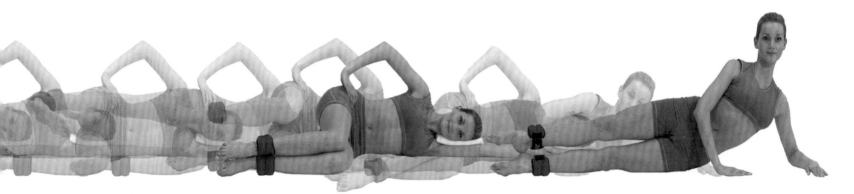

Take your right leg back to join the left leg. Be careful not to arch your back at all. Keep your abdominals engaged, your spine lengthened, and your eyes straight ahead.

● Now, slide your right leg over the left leg, and flex and point the foot. Repeat up to four times.

● Keep your right hand on your right hip and remember to keep your abdominals contracted so that your spine is supported. Then, begin to stretch both legs out so they are aligned with the rest of your body.

● Bring your right hand in front of your stomach with the palm down. Keep your heels together and rise onto your left elbow. Turn over and repeat this exercise on the other side.

diamond press

back extensors, shoulder stabilizers

This shoulder press will stretch the front of the spine and thighs as you kick. Beginners should study the first two images and attempt the leg kick with the forearms and lower ribs on the floor. Do not attempt this exercise if you have lower back or knee problems.

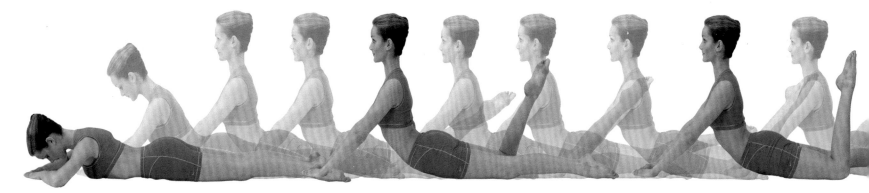

● Begin this sequence lying on your stomach, with your forehead resting on your hands and your legs outstretched, toes pointing away from the body. With your elbows extended to your sides, your arms should form a diamond shape.

● Lift your lower abs up toward your spine and push up from the palms of your hands. Continue the raise until your arms are straight and your head is facing upright. Repeat this raise three or four times. You will feel a stretch along the abdomen.

● Holding yourself up on your arms with your head facing forward, slowly raise your right foot, flexing at the knee. Keep your foot pointed toward the ceiling to form a 90 degree angle if this is comfortable.

● Now, lower the leg and repeat the exercise with the other leg, remembering to keep your foot pointed throughout the movement. Repeat the raise on both legs three or four times.

■ inhale　　exhale　Ⅱ　inhale　exhale　　▶　inhale　Ⅱ　exhale

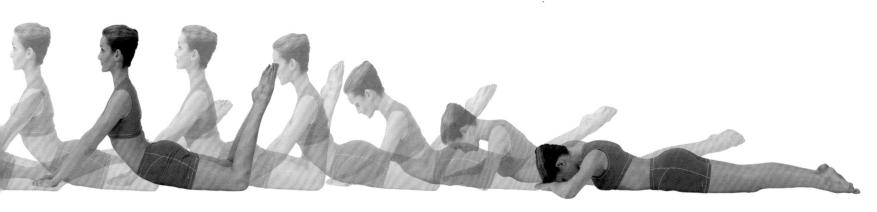

● Lower both legs back down to rest on the floor, keeping your body raised on your extended arms. Now bring both legs up together to point your toes to the ceiling. Do not bring the legs back more than feels comfortable. Keep the lower abs contracted.

● Lengthen your neck and look up a little toward the ceiling. Do not continue with this move if you feel any discomfort, especially in your lower back, knees, or neck.

● Release the stretch. Lower your head forward toward the ground, at the same time extending your legs to rest your feet on the floor.

● Bring your elbows to rest flat on the floor in the diamond position. Bring your head down to rest on the backs of your hands. Relax and breathe deeply, expand your ribs and let the spine lengthen and relax.

inhale   exhale || inhale   exhale   ▶   breathe deeply ||

intermediate **advanced**

salute, reach, and swim

spinal extensors and latissimus dorsi

A perfect workout for the back, this original Pilates exercise strengthens all the muscles along your spine and increases the mobility of your upper back (thoracic spine) and shoulder girdle. Although the lower back is extended, keep your lower abdominals contracted throughout. Think "long in the limbs" and "lifted through the center." Do not use this exercise if you have shoulder or lower back problems.

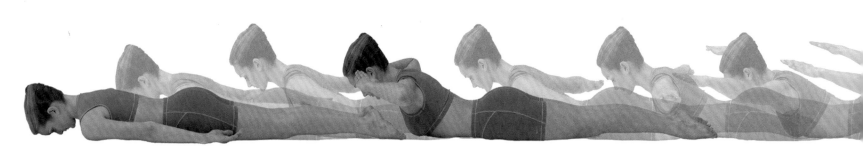

● Lie on your stomach with your forehead touching the floor and your chin tucked in. Have your arms by your side with your hands resting palms up. Lengthen your spine and pull in your abdominal muscles.

● Begin to turn your palms into your body and start to lift your head slowly. Make sure you use your abdominal muscles to lift your navel off the floor and squeeze your buttocks together a little to help keep your pelvis steady.

● Turn your palms to face the floor, keep your head up, and bring both arms up at a right angle to your head in a saluting gesture. Make sure you don't let your elbows drop. Repeat this exercise four times.

● After the fourth repetition, bring your arms back to the side of your body. Now bring the arms up in a straight line in front of you and hold the stretch. Repeat this exercise four times too.

inhale ▶ exhale inhale ▶ exhale ▶

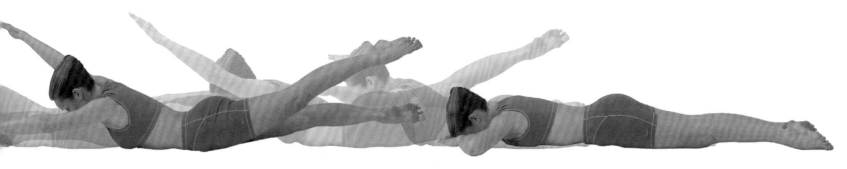

After you've finished this sequence, place your forehead on the floor again. Inhale, pulling your navel into your spine as you start to bring your right arm and your left arm up into the air simultaneously.

● If possible, lift both legs off the floor when doing this exercise. Do not lift too high—the lengthening of the limbs is more important. Lower the limbs to change to the other side. Work from your hips, not your knees.

● Keep the movement slow and controlled, making sure your arms and legs are as straight as possible. Do not allow your stomach to drop as this will put strain on your lower back. Keep your lower abs contracted.

● When you have finished, bend your elbows and put your forehead onto your arms. Keep your neck lengthened, and relax.

hamstring curls and double leg kicks

medial and lateral hamstrings

This original Pilates exercise works the buttocks (gluteals) and hamstrings, and stretches the front of the thigh (quadriceps). Aim to contract your glutes before the kick. This helps you work from the hip, not the knee. Keep you lower abdominals contracted so that your back does not overarch and your pelvis does not twist. Avoid this exercise if you have knee or lower back problems.

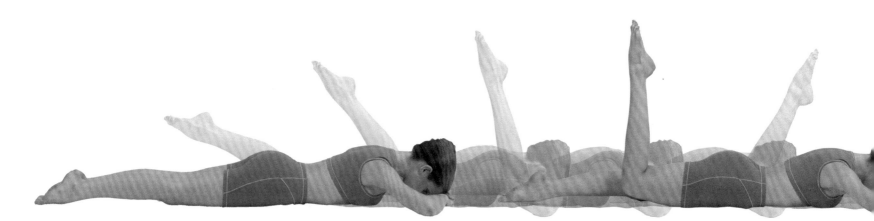

● Begin with your forehead on your fingers and your body outstretched. Take a deep breath in, contract your lower abs and lengthen the spine.

● Keeping your head in the same position, lengthen your left leg and breathe out as you begin to lift it about an inch from the floor.

● Take a breath in as you begin to bend the right knee up toward your bottom. Make sure that the opposite leg remains on the floor. Keep your stomach contracted, your shoulders relaxed, and your neck lengthened.

● Bring the leg up so that it is at a right angle to your body, if this is comfortable, and then as you breathe out, flex the foot. Breathe in, point your foot, and then bring the leg back down again. Repeat with the other leg

inhale ▶ exhale ▶ inhale ▶ exhale ▶ inhale ▶

Begin on the right leg again, ontract your lower abs, bend your nee, and bring the leg up hard to our right buttock. Take it back to a ight angle, flex the foot, and then oring it back again.

● On an out breath, lower your leg down again with your foot pointing out. Keep your upper thighs and knees glued together as you kick to engage the hamstring and buttock muscles, and help your core control.

● Repeat using the other leg. Keep your abdominal muscles contracted throughout this exercise and lengthen your body from the crown of your head so that you maintain a long neck to support the weight of your head.

● When you have finished this sequence, sit back on your heels to release your lower back. Then push back into the half cat.

exhale   inhale ▶   exhale   inhale ▶   exhale   ▶

quad and hamstring stretch

This exercise stretches the front and back of your thighs (quads and hamstrings). It is important to keep your abdominals pulled in and concentrate on keeping your back aligned in its natural curves (in neutral). Do not attempt this exercise if you have knee problems. If you have lower back problems or are a beginner, only attempt the first part of the stretch for the front of the thigh.

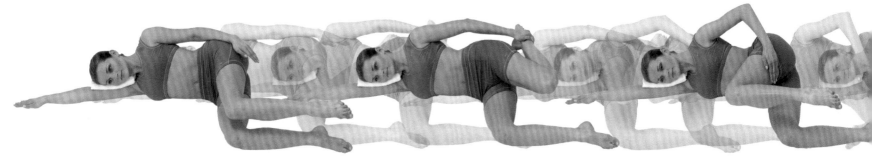

● Lie on your right side with your legs bent at a 90 degree angle. Rest your head on your right arm. You can place a pillow underneath for extra comfort. Place your left arm on your hip. Breathe in and lengthen the spine.

● Slowly lift the left leg off the floor and then begin to move it back toward your buttocks.

● Clasp your ankle with your left hand and pull your left leg back so that it is touching, or near, your buttocks. Keep your shoulders relaxed and the other knee firmly on the floor.

● Place your left hand on your left thigh and move your leg around to the front of your body.

■   ‖ inhale   ▶ exhale   ▶ inhale   ▶

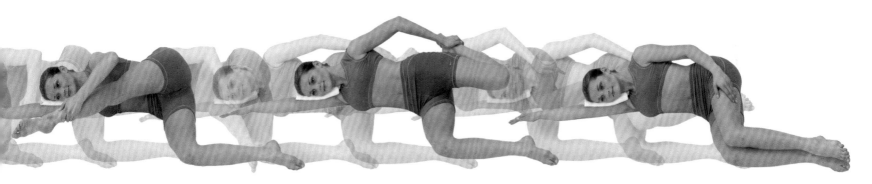

Start to straighten the left leg out in front of you, moving your hand up for support. Pull the straight leg up as far as possible. Contract your lower abs and only pull the leg as far as you can feel a comfortable stretch.

● Now, move your left leg back toward your right leg, bending the knee as you do so. Keep your chest open and your shoulders relaxed as you perform this exercise.

● Bend the leg back toward your buttocks, as before. Grip your ankle with your left hand and feel the stretch all along your thigh. Keep your lower abs pulled in and do not allow your spine to overarch.

● Allow your left leg to rest on your right leg again. Pause and repeat the exercise up to four times. Then, turn onto your left side and follow the same sequence on the other side. Repeat up to four times.

ballet legs

gluteals and adductors

The combined movements of this exercise stretch and strengthen all the major muscles in the legs and hips. The sequence also challenges your core stability as the legs stretch out. Beginners should only take the leg to 45 degrees and bend the supporting leg. Do not attempt this exercise if you have knee or lower back problems.

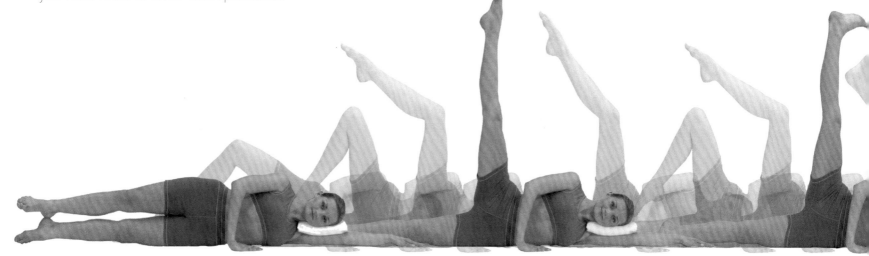

● Begin the exercise by lying on your left side with your head resting on your arm. You can use a pillow if this is uncomfortable. Put your other arm in front of your body with the hand flat on the floor.

● With your body in a line through your shoulders, hips, and knees, lift your right leg up, drawing an imaginary line with your toes along you left leg. Beginners should bring their knee to 45 degrees, others to 90 degrees.

● When you reach 45 or 90 degrees, flex the foot and put it down in front of the left leg. Push your right leg up again as far as you can toward your head, and then place it back down again and point both toes together.

● Breathe in and bring your turned out foot toward your knee. Then breathe out as you straighten the leg to the ceiling.

inhale ▶ exhale ▶ inhale exhale ▶

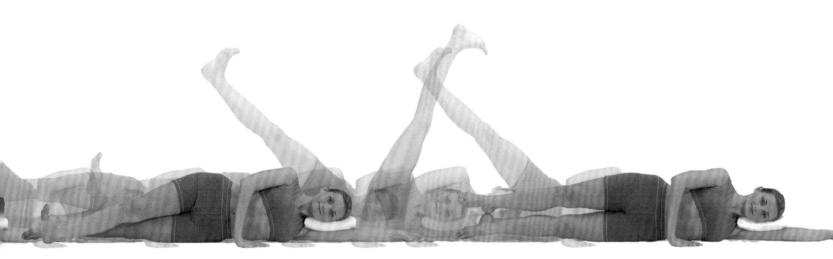

● Breathe in as you flex the foot. Push with the heel and maintain a long leg and foot. Then reverse the motion and lower the leg to the floor, keeping your pelvis steady.

● Breathe out and lengthen the leg as before, then breathe in to lift it back up again. Keep your leg straight and your foot flexed. Be careful not to sink into your shoulder or waist as you straighten your leg to the ceiling.

● Lift your top leg as far back as is comfortable. Concentrate on maintaining a long and stable torso as you perform this sequence and don't allow your knee, thigh, or foot to roll inward.

● Breathe out and begin to lower the leg back down again. Keep your leg lengthened and controlled. End this exercise in the same position as you started. Turn over and repeat the exercise on the other side.

inhale ▶ exhale inhale ▶ begin to exhale ▶ exhale

intro to 100s

abdominal muscles

This original Pilates exercise is excellent for strengthening your abdominal muscles. It is important to maintain a neutral spine when the feet are on the floor. Beginners should study the first three images and keep the feet down, using one hand to support the head, before progressing. If you have neck or lower back problems, try the beginners version but stop if you feel any strain.

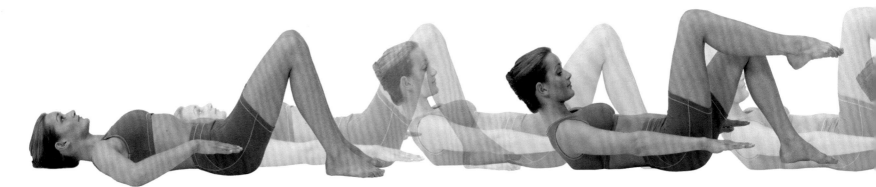

● Start on your back with your knees bent. Have your arms slightly bent and raised level with your ribs. Breathe in and lengthen your spine. Then breathe in and out five times, focusing on hollowing your abdominals.

● Now stretch your arms out beside you, reaching from deep in the pit of your arm as if you were trying to touch a wall on the other side of the room with your fingertips.

● Lift your head up to look at your navel. Make sure you are bending forward from your upper torso and not your neck. Keep the shoulders down, pressing away from your ears so that you stretch the neck.

● When your head is lifted up, raise your right leg up to a 90 degree angle. Keep it bent at the knee with your toes pointed out.

■ **inhale and exhale x 5**   ‖ **inhale**   ▶ **exhale**   ▶ **inhale**   ▶

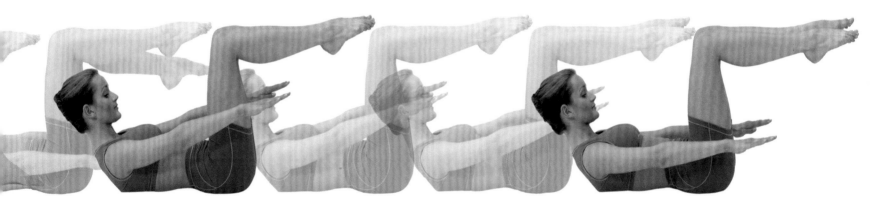

Bring your left leg up to join the right one. Focus on the weight of your stomach as it sinks into your spine, and keep your shoulder blades pressed into the floor.

● Raise both your arms to a 45 degree angle. Maintain your back position on the mat, hollowing your abdominals and not allowing your back to arch.

● You can place a small pillow or rolled towel under your head to give your neck support if you find it too difficult to keep your head lifted throughout this routine.

● Bring your arms back down again, and end by lowering your head and placing the soles of your feet back on the floor again. Remember to keep contracting your lower abs throughout this sequence.

leg dances

hip flexors and adductors

The dance movement works the lower abdominal muscles
(internal obliques), and the double leg reach works the inner
thighs (adductors) and stretches the hamstrings. Beginners can
keep their toes on the floor, dropping their knees left and right.
Do not attempt this exercise if you have lower back problems.

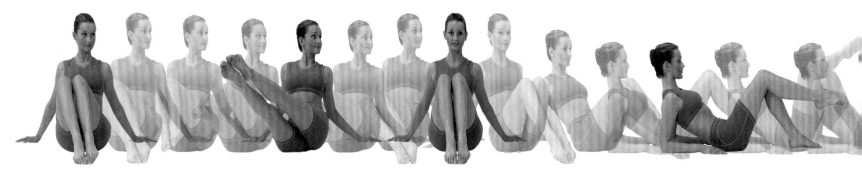

● Start by sitting upright. Support
yourself with your arms and have your
knees bent with your feet pointed out.
Begin to lean your knees to the right.

● Extend your legs at this angle, with
your head facing in the opposite
direction. Make sure that you keep
your chest lifted (don't let it sink).
Keep your arms as straight as you
can without locking the elbows.

● Take your legs back to the center
again and twist to the other side while
looking in the opposite direction again.
Repeat these extensions between two
and four times on each side.

● Now bend your arms at the elbow
and rest on your forearms. Keep your
neck long. Bend your left knee and
start to lift your right leg up into the
air. Keep your back supported by
engaging your lower abs.

inhale ▶ exhale ▶ inhale exhale ▶ begin to inhale ▶

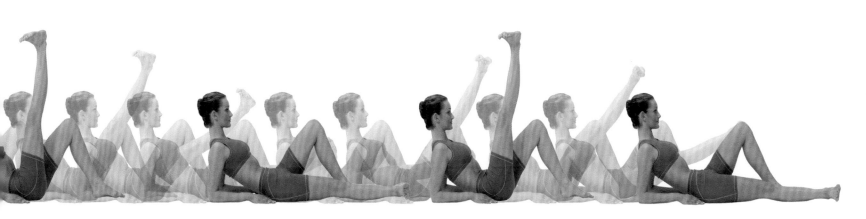

Turn your leg outward as you lift it up. Keep your toes pointed and then flex your foot when your leg is straight in front of you.

● Slowly lower your leg back down onto the floor again, keeping the leg straight and your foot turned outward. Keep your abdominal muscles pulled in tight for support.

● Breathe in and raise your leg up into the air again with the foot still turned out. Only lift it to a 90 degree angle if this is comfortable (you should not feel any strain in your lower back).

● Repeat the exercise with the other leg. Keep your ribs rolled forward and your legs controlled as you raise and lower them. Finish by uncurling to the relaxation position and breathe deeply.

advanced mermaid *quadratus lumborum*

This movement is in two parts—a beginners and an advanced Mermaid pose. The

sequence stretches and strengthens the muscles of the shoulders, arms, and side of the

spine. Beginners should practice the seated pose before progressing. Do not attempt the

second part of this exercise if you have neck, shoulder, or wrist problems.

● Begin the sequence sitting upright, with your legs tucked under your body but to one side. Keeping your left hand on the floor, raise your right arm and extend outward so that the arm is parallel with your shoulder.

● Continue to raise your arm and rotate the hand so that the palm is facing inward toward your body. Bend the arm at the elbow to form a gentle curve so that the palm is facing down toward your head.

● With your left hand flat on the floor, lower your body sideway toward the floor. Bend your arm to bring it down and rest on your elbow. Keep your right arm in the same pose throughout so that the palm is now facing down toward the floor.

● Pushing with the left hand, raise your body to sit upright, with your feet still tucked to one side. Once you are sitting upright, lower your right arm and raise your left hand in a smooth flowing movement. Your abdominals should be contracted throughout.

■ **inhale** **exhale** ▶ **inhale** ‖ **exhale** ▶

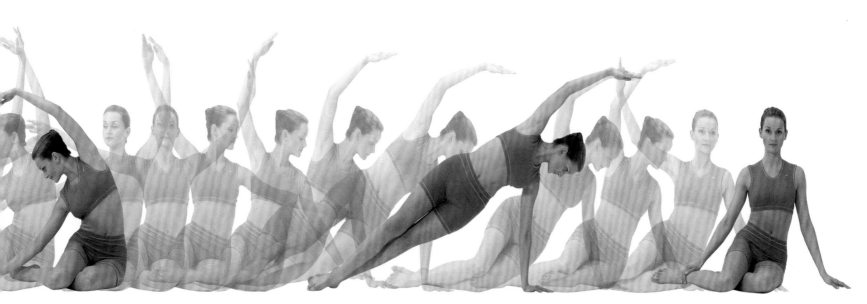

Now, bend your body to the right, ringing your right hand down to rest your right foot. At the same time, ce toward the right and raise your ft arm. Rotate the palm inward so at the palm extends beyond your ad and faces down to the floor.

● Now, raise your body back to the center and face forward with both arms extended. Then, gently lower yourself to the left until your left hand is pressed palm down onto the floor. Slowly extend your legs out from under your body.

● With your head turned down to your left, push your feet into the floor to bring your body upright. Extend your left arm to lock at the elbow and extend your legs out fully. Extend your right arm over your head so that the palm is facing down to the floor.

● Imagine you are suspended at the hips by a sling attached to the ceiling. Hold the pose briefly. Now lower your body back down to the start position. Rest your arms, relax, breathe deeply, and expand your chest. Now, do the exercise on the other side.

hale ▶ exhale inhale ‖ exhale ▶ ‖

half cat and ankle stretch *and tibialis anterior*

The half cat stretches the back and shoulder muscles (spinal extensors and latissimus dorsi).

The knee raise stretches the muscles that run along the front of the lower leg (tibialis anterior).

Do not attempt to press your chest to the floor as shown in the sequence—this is for advanced

exercisers only. Do not attempt this exercise if you have knee problems.

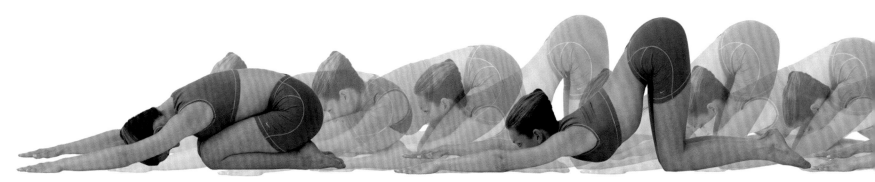

● Start by sitting on your heels with your knees tucked under your body and your forehead resting on the floor. Your arms should be fully extended but relaxed. Breathe in and lengthen your spine.

● Lift your head up about six to eight inches (15–20 cm). Keep your neck lengthened and then creep forward, lowering your chest to the floor and raising your hips in the air.

● Make sure that your upper legs are vertical and your spine is lengthened as you stretch your upper body.

● Now, scoop your lower abdominal in, tuck your bottom under, and slide back to sit on your heels again. Repeat this exercise slowly and carefully four times.

‖ inhale   ▶ exhale   ▶ inhale   exhale▶

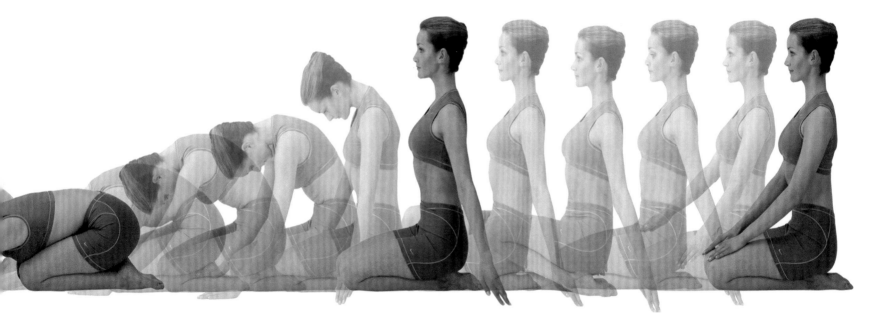

After you have finished the four stretches, begin to sit up on your feet. Curl your back and gradually lift your neck up too. Slide your hands back as you raise your chest.

● As you sit up straight, bring your hands to your sides with the fingertips resting on the floor.

● Raise the right knee off the floor a few inches. You can lean slightly back as you do this movement. Put the knee back down again and repeat with the left knee.

● Raise your knees alternately four times each, then bring your hands forward into your lap and rest them on your knees.

inhale ▶ exhale inhale ❚❚ ▶ ❚❚

final release

cat and table legs *pelvic and shoulder girdle stability*

This exercise will strengthen your back muscles and improve

spinal flexibility. The "cat" stretches your upper back and

shoulders while the leg and arm stretches challenge your core

control and hip and shoulder flexibility. If you suffer from knee,

shoulder, or wrist problems, approach this exercise with caution.

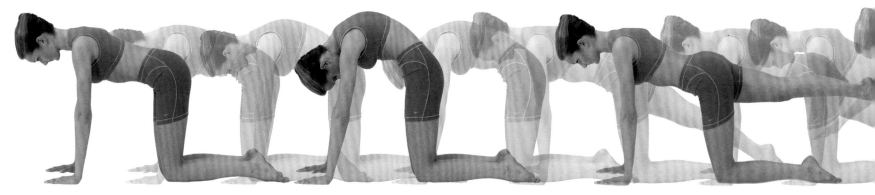

● Begin this exercise kneeling on all fours keeping the long shallow curves of your spine in the neutral position. Be careful not to put too much pressure on your wrists—if you feel any pain, stop.

● Slowly begin to arch your back up. Curl from the pelvis and lengthen your neck. Keep your arms and legs still to support this movement. Release, straighten your back, and repeat four times.

● Now, lengthen your right leg to its full extent and raise it to a 90 degree angle. Make sure you keep your hips aligned as you do this sequence.

● Bring your leg back down again. Repeat the exercise using the other leg. Keep looking down at the floor and don't let your head and neck drop. Only lift your leg as high as you can keep your pelvis square.

| ■ inhale | exhale | ‖ inhale | exhale | ▶ inhale | ▶ |

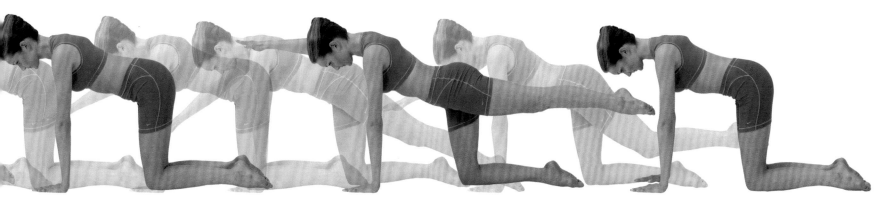

Keeping your pelvis square, your spine lengthened, and your shoulders relaxed, lift the right arm forward toward a 90 degree angle. Beginners should keep the arm in a low "salute."

● Bring the arm slowly down again and repeat this exercise with the other arm. Make sure you don't twist from the hips. Keep your neck long, your back flat, and your lower abdominals pulled into your spine.

● Now, combine the arm and leg movements. Begin with your left leg and right arm, and raise them both slowly. Keep your shoulders down and concentrate on lengthening the spine and pulling in the lower abdominals.

● Lower your arms and legs to the floor again, and then repeat this movement with your right leg and left arm.

advanced table legs

This exercise is named the "table," as this image helps remind you to keep your hips and shoulders horizontal as you work through the stretch. The leg and arm reach works your hip and shoulder muscles, and tests your balance and core control. Do not attempt this exercise if you have knee, shoulder, or lower back problems.

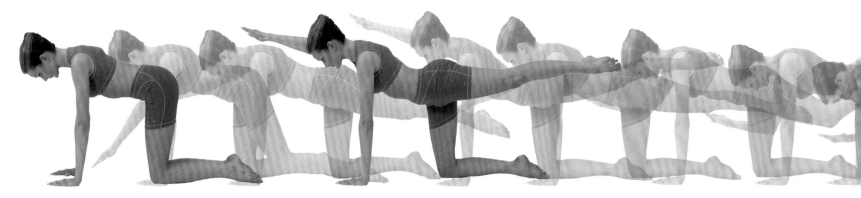

● Kneel forward and place your hands under your shoulders with your fingers facing forward. Have your back straight, your knees at a right angle to your body, and look down at the floor. Breathe in and lengthen the spine.

● Contract your lower abdominals and extend your left leg and right arm at the same time. If you have a strong center (a balance of good abdominals and back muscles) you can continue to stretch your limbs a little further.

● Breathe in and then on a breath out, bring your leg and arm down again, and start to bend your knee in toward your body. Keep your neck lengthened and your supporting leg and arm steady.

● Taking care not to twist your body as you move your leg, start to bend your head in toward your knee. Make sure your shoulders are not hunched and that your lower abdominals keep working.

■   ‖ exhale   ▶   inhale   exhale   inhale   ▶

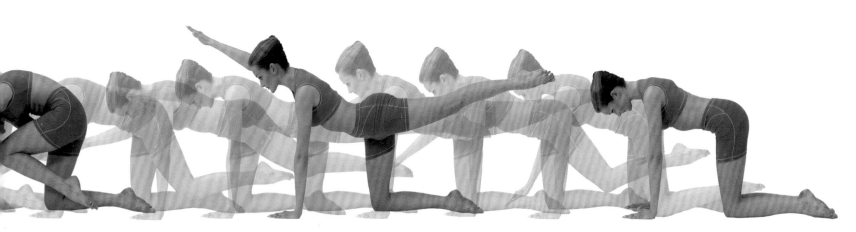

● Bring your knee up to your chin and your right elbow bent into the side of your body. Keep your stomach followed throughout this sequence and your shoulders down.

● Start to extend your right arm and your left leg again. Remember that most people stop this movement when their limbs are horizontal. Only attempt to raise your limbs higher if you are at an advanced level.

● Hold the pose briefly and then take your arm and leg back down toward your torso again.

● Finish this part of the exercise on all fours as you did at the beginning. Then, repeat the sequence on the other side, stretching the left arm and the right leg.

begin to exhale   ▶ exhale   inhale   ‖   ▶   ‖

lateral raise with arm weights

This exercise will strengthen your back and shoulder muscles (rhomboids, latissimus dorsi, trapezius, and deltoids). Beginners should practice sitting on a chair leaning forward to a 30 degree angle. If you have shoulder or back problems try the sitting version, but stop if you feel any discomfort.

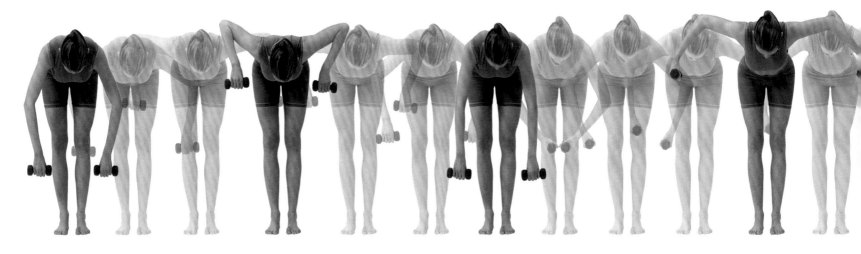

● Begin standing up. Bend over at the waist so your body is at a 90 degree angle. Imagine your back is as flat as a table with your shoulders open and not hunched. Have your arms loose and palms facing back.

● Keep your feet parallel and bend the elbows up as far as you can. Make sure your knees are bent slightly and that your hands keep facing down.

● Lower your arms back down again, making sure your head remains aligned with your spine and does not hang forward at all. Repeat this exercise. Keep your lower abdominals pulled in to support your back.

● Now, bend your elbows out to the sides so that they are parallel to your shoulders, or slightly higher, and repeat. Make sure this is a slow and controlled movement.

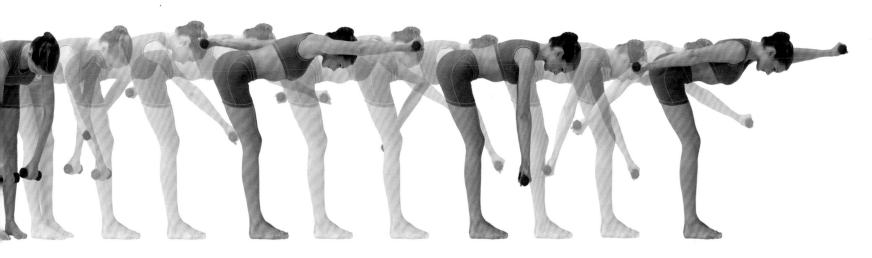

Breathe out as you bring your arms together. Now, inhale and simultaneously extend your right arm straight out in front of you and the other arm straight behind you.

● Be careful not to throw your arms forward or back. All movements should be slow and controlled with the deeper abdominal muscles pulling in around the waist throughout the exercise.

● Exhale and bring your arms back in front of you again. Keep the shoulders down and your abdomen engaged. If your back hurts at any point during this exercise, stop immediately.

● Inhale as you repeat the sequence with the opposite arm leading. Make sure your extended arms are parallel to your body. Repeat up to eight times.

exhale   inhale ▶   begin to exhale   ▶   exhale   ▶   inhale

roll ups with pole abdominals, hip flexors, and vertebrae

The roll up is an original Pilates exercise that stretches all the muscles along the back of your body, articulates the spine, and strengthens your abdominals, which can help flatten the stomach. The pole is used to help keep your arms parallel and shoulders level. Beginners should only roll up half way, keeping the knees bent. Do not do this exercise if you have lower back or shoulder problems.

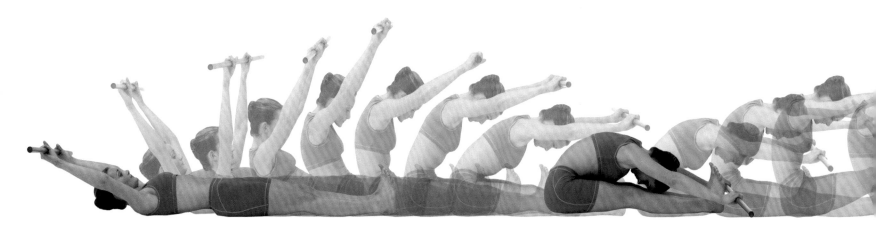

- Lie on your back and lengthen your body. Your arms should be straight behind your head. Have your palms facing up and your feet flexed. Hollow your lower abdominals by pulling them into your spine.

- Squeeze your buttocks tightly and press the back of your upper inner thighs together. Begin to raise your arms straight up, bringing your head, neck, and back up, too. Inhale as you begin to roll up and forward.

- Be careful not to let your legs lift off the mat as you roll up. Fold all the way forward as far as you can, then breathe out as you stretch forward from the hips while keeping your stomach pulled back into your spine.

- Start to roll down by squeezing your buttocks together and slightly tucking your tailbone underneath you. Breathe in as you begin pulling your stomach into your spine again.

inhale   inhale ▶   exhale ▶   inhale ▶

● Breathe out as you bend your
knees and begin to roll back down.
Feel each vertebra pressing into the
floor as you descend slowly and
carefully, keeping your lower
abdominals drawn in toward them.

● Keep squeezing the back of your
upper inner thighs together for
stability, and keep your chin tucked
into your chest so you are not pulling
from the neck.

● Concentrate on lengthening the
spine as you do this exercise. Keep the
lower body still, and focus on the
spinal muscles.

● When the back of your shoulders
touch the floor, lower your head and
bring your arms over it. Stretch your
body out fully, then repeat the
exercise between four and eight times.

teaser abdominals and hip flexors

This original Pilates exercise is a demanding workout for the abdominals and hip muscles. It also challenges your core control and your balance as you coordinate arms and legs. Beginners can try the version shown up to one leg raise. Do not attempt this exercise if you have lower back or neck problems.

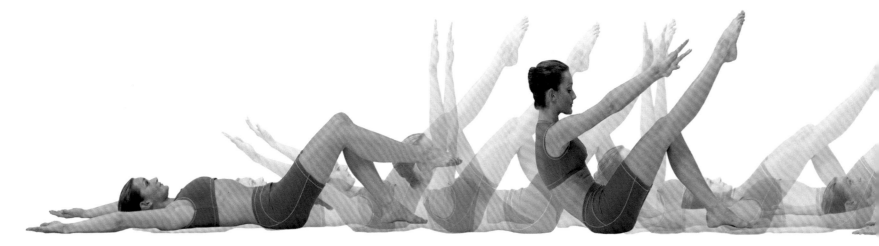

● Start this exercise lying on your back with your arms straight out above your head. Hollow your lower abdominals in toward the spine and press your lower back gently into the mat without tucking.

● Breathe in and lengthen the spine. Breathe out and straighten your right leg up to a 45 degree angle. Press the knees together. Hold your leg in this position and squeeze your buttocks and inner thighs together tightly.

● Now, raise your arms above your head and allow your head and upper body to begin to lift from the floor, too. Reach your hands toward your outstretched toes, and lift out of your waist as you breathe in.

● As you breathe out, begin to roll your spine slowly back down on the floor. Keep your right leg up in the air, and stretch your arms back over your head. Beginners can roll back down and repeat with the other leg.

inhale ‖ exhale inhale ▶ exhale ▶

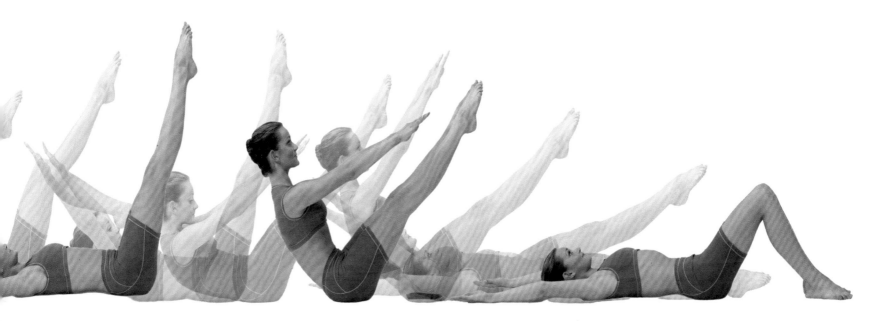

● Now, bring the left leg up to join the other leg. Keep your toes pointed and make sure you maintain a flat and stable back.

● Lower your legs to a 45 degree angle. Inhale, bring your arms over your head and reach toward your toes, creating a V shape. Balancing on your tailbone, hold this pose with your abdominals pulled into your spine.

● Breathe out as you begin rolling your spine back down onto the floor again. Squeeze your buttocks to help keep your pelvis stable and support the weight of your legs.

● When your head touches the floor, stretch your arms out over your head again and bend your knees. Repeat this whole sequence up to five times as your stamina and strength improves.

exhale ▶ inhale ‖ exhale ▶ inhale ■

chalk circles

pectoralis major

This exercise mobilizes the spine and stretches your pectoral muscles, helping to release tension in your shoulders and upper back. It is a gentle exercise, but you should still approach it carefully if you have any spinal problems. You can repeat this exercise up to 10 times.

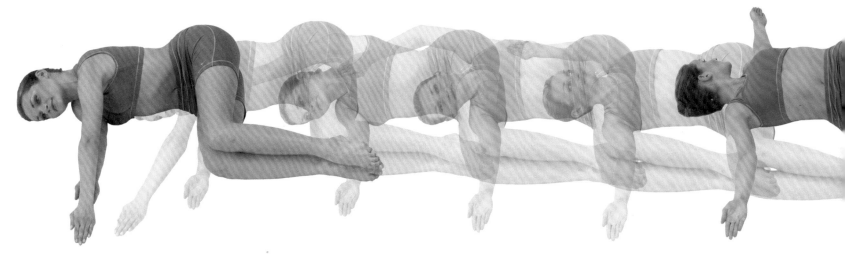

● Start by lying on your right side with your legs bent at the knee at a 90 degree angle to your body. Put your hands together with your arms straight out in front of you. If your neck hurts, place a pillow under it.

● Breathe out and begin to slowly move your left arm along the floor toward the top of your head.

● Stretch your arm over your head, keeping your fingers on the floor if possible. Imagine you are drawing a wide circle with a piece of chalk as you circle your arm over to the other side of your head.

● Breathe out as you open your chest and turn your head toward your left arm, relaxing as best as you can. Hold this position and then take a deep breath in visualizing your chest opening and stretching.

■ inhale   ‖ exhale   ▶ inhale   ▶ exhale   ‖ inhale

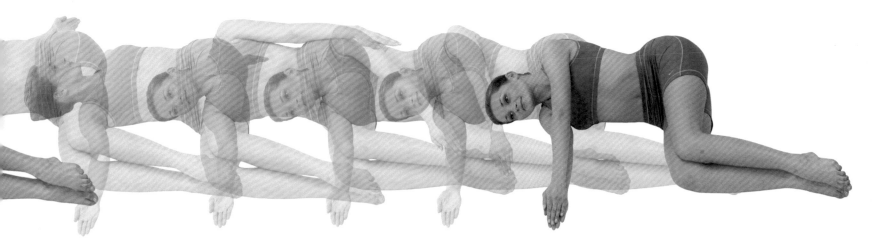

● Breathe out, tighten your stomach muscles, and then start to move your left arm in a circle down toward your buttocks. Bend your elbow if this is more comfortable.

● Stretch your arm out and move your palm down, as you pass your hip—this will give your neck a good stretch. Keep your abdominal muscles engaged to support your back.

● Breathe in as you place your hands together to complete the circle. Keep your knees at a 90 degree angle at all times to avoid straining your lower back.

● Repeat this exercise four times, then lie on your left side and follow the same circular movement with your right arm.

exhale   ▷ exhale   inhale   ‖   ▷   ‖

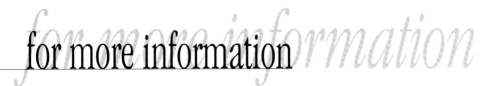

IDEA Health & Fitness Association

10455 Pacific Center Court

San Diego, CA 92121

(858) 535-8979

Web site: http://www.ideafit.com

Organization that provides fitness professionals with resources and information about the fitness industry.

Medical Fitness Association

P.O. Box 73103

Richmond, VA 23235-8026

(804) 897-5701

Web site: http://www.medicalfitness.org

Nonprofit organization working to develop and operate medically integrated fitness centers.

Pilates Method Alliance

P.O. Box 370906

Miami, FL 33137-0906

(866) 573-4945

Web site: http://www.pilatesmethodalliance.org

Association that establishes certification and standards for Pilates professionals.

President's Council on Physical Fitness and Sports

Department W

Tower Building, Suite 560

1101 Wootton Parkway

Rockville, MD 20852

(240) 276-9567
Web site: http://www.fitness.gov
An advisory committee of volunteer citizens who advise the president through the secretary of health and human services about physical activity, fitness, and sports in America.

U.S. Department of Health and Human Services
200 Independence Avenue SW
Washington, DC 20201
(877) 696-6775
Web site: http://www.hhs.gov
The U.S. government's principal agency for protecting the health of all Americans and providing essential human services.

YMCA of the USA
101 North Wacker Drive
Chicago, IL 60606
(800) 872-9622
Web site: http://www.ymca.net
Nonprofit community service organization working toward building strength within communities and promoting physical fitness.

Web Sites

Due to the changing nature of Internet links, Rosen Publishing has developed an online list of Web sites related to the subject of this book. This site is updated regularly. Please use this link to access the list:

http://www.rosenlinks.com/sim/pila

for further reading

Daniels, Diane. *Pilates Perfect: The Complete Guide to Pilates Exercise at Home.* New York, NY: Random House, 2004.

Ellsworth, Abby. *Pilates Anatomy.* Charlotte, NC: Thunder Bay, 2009.

Herdman, Alan. *The Pilates Directory.* New York, NY: Metro Books, 2009.

Herman, Ellie. *Ellie Herman's Pilates Props Workbook.* Berkeley, CA: Ulysses, 2004.

Isacowitz, Rael. *Pilates: Your Complete Guide to Mat Work and Apparatus Exercises.* Champaign, IL: Human Kinetics, 2006.

Keane, Sandie. *Pilates for Core Strength.* Delafield, WI: Main Street Press, 2005.

Lyon, Daniel. *Complete Book of Pilates for Men: The Lifetime Plan for Strength, Power and Peak Performance.* New York, NY: HarperCollins, 2005.

Massey, Paul. *Anatomy of Pilates.* Berkeley, CA: North Atlantic, 2009.

Monks, Jonathan, and Emily Kelly. *Pilates Yoga.* London, UK: Anness, 2004.

Siler, Brooke. *Your Ultimate Pilates Body Challenge: At the Gym, on the Mat, and on the Move.* New York, NY: Broadway Books, 2005.

Smith, Judy, Emily Kelly, and Jonathan Monks. *Pilates and Yoga.* New York, NY: Metro Books, 2006.

Ungaro, Alycea. *15 Minute Everyday Pilates.* New York, NY: DK, 2007.

Worth, Yvonne. *Pilates.* London, UK: HarperCollins UK, 2004.

about the author

Dr. Louise Aikman is an editor and author of many nonfiction books.

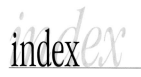